Interface:

Explore a groundbreaking approach to managing diabetes with "Intermittent Fasting for Diabetes." In this comprehensive guide, you'll embark on a transformative journey toward better health and improved blood sugar control. Discover the power of harnessing your body's natural rhythms through intermittent fasting, a scientifically proven method that has the potential to revolutionize diabetes management.

Within these pages, you'll delve into the science behind intermittent fasting and how it can positively impact your diabetes. Learn about various fasting protocols and how to tailor them to your unique needs, ensuring a safe and effective approach. Say goodbye to restrictive diets and hello to a flexible and sustainable way of eating that aligns with your diabetes management goals.

This book doesn't just stop at the basics; it provides practical tips, meal plans, and delicious recipes designed to make intermittent fasting a seamless part of your lifestyle. Whether you're newly diagnosed or have been living with diabetes for years, "Intermittent Fasting for Diabetes" offers a comprehensive roadmap to better blood sugar control, improved insulin sensitivity, and enhanced overall well-being.

Take control of your diabetes journey today and unlock the potential for a healthier, more vibrant life through the transformative power of intermittent fasting.

Table of Contents

Chapter 1:

Introduction

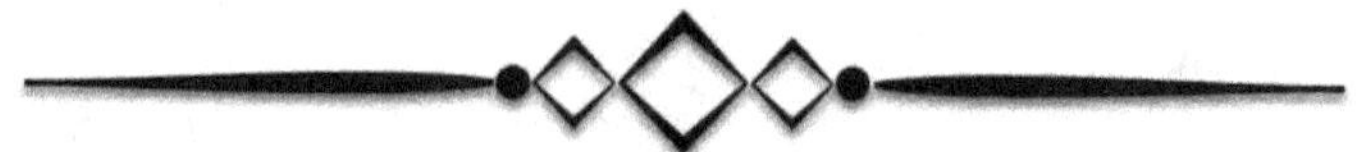

ntermittent fasting has become a popular topic among those seeking to control their health and well-being. With the worry around worldwide diabetes rates growing, it is not surprising that this dietary trend has gained attention from individuals searching for alternatives to customary weight-loss approaches. Intermittent fasting consists of cycles where people alternate between consuming meals and abstaining from them; research indicates that it may have multiple potential benefits for diabetic management, including enhancing blood glucose level regulation, increasing insulin sensitivity, and reducing cholesterol amounts.

Understanding of intermittent fasting on diabetes management

Considerable research has been devoted to exploring the potential benefits of intermittent fasting on diabetes management. Intermittent fasting is an approach whereby food consumption is limited for up to 24 hours. One promising use associated with this practice appears to be its capacity for reducing insulin resistance and consequently enhancing glycemic control in persons who have type 2 diabetes. Additionally, when performed correctly, intermittent fasting can lead to weight loss and enhanced blood glucose levels; furthermore, it has demonstrated effectiveness similar to traditional calorie-restricted diets in achieving these objectives. Further studies have suggested that periodic abstinence from eating may reduce risk factors leading to cardiovascular disease and other medical issues such as hypertension or dyslipidemia-connected chronic ailments. Some experts even assert that well-being might be additionally boosted using intermittent fasting by reducing inflammation within the body, improving sleep quality, increasing mental clarity, and inspiring positive emotional states. Consequently, understanding the likely advantages of sporadic abstaining could significantly aid in managing type 2 diabetes.

Exploring the science behind Intermittent Fasting

Intermittent fasting, often referred to as IF for short, is a dietary approach that consists of alternating periods of consuming and abstaining from food. Research has found this method helpful in weight loss, overall health benefits, and the management of certain chronic diseases such as diabetes. Despite its potential advantages for those with diabetes specifically, one must understand the science behind how intermittent fasting operates so they can make informed decisions concerning their well-being.

Research into the influence of intermittent fasting on individuals with diabetes is still in progress. Several studies, especially those that seem to have potential, signify that IF could aid in enhancing insulin sensitivity and diminishing blood sugar levels for people with type 2 diabetes [1].

However, many things remain yet to be explored within this field of study – including understanding how different types of IF may affect distinct people differently.

A central aspect when comprehending how intermittent fasting impacts people with diabetes is the timing during which meals and snacks are consumed. Consuming too few calories or eating at irregular periods can lead to disruption in glucose regulation levels.

Research suggests that those with diabetes who wish to try intermittent fasting (IF) must consume consistent daily calories to maintain stable glucose levels. Moreover, leaving lengthy gaps between meals can result in postprandial hypoglycemia – or low blood sugar [2].

Furthermore, individuals should take into consideration diet composition when considering IF and type 2 diabetes management[3], avoiding foods high in sugar, which could lead to significant increases in glucose levels, and instead opting for more slowly digested whole grains, skinny proteins, and healthy fats; this will help minimize drastic peaks or troughs of their blood sugar levels. Numerous factors require substantial deliberation before making decisions regarding the science behind intermittent fasting and its potential effects on people with diabetes; however, appropriately executing such an approach may benefit those with type 2 diabetes.

Potential benefits of Intermittent Fasting for general health

Upon examining the potential advantages of intermittent fasting for overall health, this particular dietary pattern may yield many laudable outcomes. Research has indicated an association between intermittent fasting and reduced susceptibility to obesity, type 2 diabetes, cancer, heart disease, and stroke. Observing fasts at certain intervals during a day or week can reduce caloric intake, which results in weight reduction. Additionally, engaging in such practices at appropriate times allows the body to enter into ketosis, a state with more fat-burning and improved metabolic processes.

Additionally, intermittent fasting may reduce inflammation levels in the body through its effects on metabolic hormones such as insulin and ghrelin. It benefits those with existing inflammation-related conditions, including arthritis or other autoimmune diseases. Furthermore, research indicates that intermittent fasting can also impact neurodegenerative diseases like Alzheimer's by increasing the production of brain-derived neurotrophic factor, which is essential for cognitive and memory functions.

In addition, one might experience improved mental health from engaging in this practice due to better sleep quality and lower stress levels. Consequently, it stands to reason why many individuals choose intermittent fasting as a viable option for improving their overall well-being without having to make dramatic lifestyle modifications or resorting to excessive dieting practices.

How Intermittent Fasting Can Benefit Individuals with Diabetes?

Intermittent fasting, a way of dieting that alternates between consuming and abstaining from food, has become an effective means of weight loss. However, the effects it may have on diabetes are now beginning to be realized. Recent studies have indicated that people with diabetes can gain multiple advantages from intermittent fasting, primarily by improving their blood sugar regulation. It is necessary to point out that those with diabetes should consult their physician before attempting this eating regimen since certain forms of the diet could not be apt for individuals with precise medical issues.

Regarding Type 1 Diabetes, research has indicated that fasting may diminish postprandial or after-meal glucose levels without augmenting the jeopardy of hypoglycemia or low blood sugar. It implies that those with Type 1 Diabetes might include a fasting period into their daily regimen to lessen peak blood glucose concentrations following meals. Additionally, it is possible that abstaining from food could also facilitate an improvement in sensitivity towards insulin - which functions as the hormone responsible for controlling blood sugar - potentially delivering supplementary assistance when managing symptoms associated with Type 1 Diabetes.

For those with Type 2 Diabetes, intermittent fasting is more practical in controlling blood sugar levels than traditional caloric restriction diets. Recent evidence further suggests that alternating activity patterns between days and prolonged periods of overnight fasting can lead to increased physical movement and improved sleep quality - both paramount components for managing the symptoms of Type 2 Diabetes.

The potential health advantages associated with intermittent fasting are encouraging; however, conclusive information about its efficacy in diabetic patients cannot be determined until further research is conducted. Nevertheless, the data appears promising, which could open up new paths for individuals searching for ways to manage their condition while improving overall health outcomes effectively.

The Prevalence of Diabetes

Diabetes is a medical illness that can be prevented and managed, yet it affects an estimated 422 million individuals worldwide. While Type 1 diabetes accounts for only approximately 5-10% of all cases due to being caused by autoimmune devastation of insulin-producing beta cells in the pancreas, Type 2 diabetes constitutes up to 90%. This type tends to manifest among those who are older or obese/physically inactive.

Gestational Diabetes is another form that influences pregnant women specifically and has been linked with long-term health problems affecting both mother and baby alike. To regulate blood glucose levels effectively, persons who have diabetes must ensure they adhere to frequent healthcare monitoring sessions along with lifestyle changes as well as medication regimens. In recent years, researchers have considered intermittent fasting may provide some help when managing symptoms related to this disease whereby caloric intake would temporarily cease over periods ranging anywhere from one day up to multiple days per week - findings suggest this method might bring about lower rates on fasting blood glucose thereby benefitting people battling Diabetes.

Why Diabetes Matters?

Diabetes is a severe and growing global health concern, with individuals living with the condition needing to engage in life-long diligence and care for successful management. While multiple potential options are available for managing diabetes, such as dietary adjustments or medication use, intermittent fasting (IF) has emerged as an evidence-backed strategy that is gaining favor amongst people with diabetes seeking better control of their disease. Though IF cannot be said to cure or prevent diabetes, its consistent implementation may result in favorable outcomes for those living with chronic illness.

For starters, Intermittent Fasting (IF) has been demonstrated in a few studies to have beneficial effects on glycemic control and support weight loss - both advantageous for individuals with diabetes endeavoring to manage their blood sugar levels. Furthermore, IF is also known to enhance cholesterol levels, minimize inflammation throughout the body, and augment energy levels – making it an adequate tool for coping with fatigue related to diabetes daily. Moreover, there may be implications regarding mental well-being; some research suggests that IF might decrease stress hormones like cortisol, which can detrimentally affect diabetic control if left unchecked. Ultimately, this makes IF an attractive option deserving further exploration by those searching for alternative means of maintaining health while living with diabetes.

Historical background of Intermittent Fasting

The practice of intermittent fasting can be traced back to archaic cultures, where it was used as a spiritual ritual for purification. Ancient Greek philosophers thought reducing food intake could improve mental clarity and physical health. Hippocrates also believed that regular fasting had beneficial effects on general health and well-being, going so far as to recommend it as one way of treating medical conditions such as diabetes. Nowadays, adherents who observe fasts during holy days keep this tradition alive, while modern science is beginning to appreciate the potential benefits that intermittent fasting may bring people with diabetes. As part of their investigation into short-term periods with reduced calorie or carbohydrate intake's influence over glucose metabolism, insulin sensitivity, and body fat percentage in humans and animals alike - researchers have generated preliminary studies suggesting these changes might help maintain blood sugar levels amongst those who have Type 2 Diabetes more effectively. For us to gain a better understanding of how long-term impacts on diabetic patients are affected by intermittent fasting, however - further research must still be carried out.

Risks associated with Intermittent Fasting for diabetics

Fasting can be a productive means of keeping healthy and managing blood sugar levels for individuals with diabetes. Intermittent fasting, sometimes called IF, is a kind of fasting that generally involves enduring long periods without eating anything. Despite this form of diet having displayed its effectiveness for certain people, it might not necessarily be the optimum alternative for every diabetic person. Before commencing any fasting regimen, it is essential to comprehend the potential hazards associated with intermittent fasting when dealing with diabetics.

One of the significant dangers connected with intermittent fasting for people with diabetes is hypoglycemia or low blood sugar. It happens when the body does not possess enough glucose in its system to preserve customary blood sugar levels. It can lead to extreme lethargy, disarray, and even convulsions. To reduce the danger of acquiring hypoglycemia while practicing IF, people with diabetes should carefully monitor their food intake and blood glucose concentrations throughout the day and ensure they consume regularly throughout their fasting. Another potential hazard is putting on weight caused by over-eating after a period of abstaining from food.

When it comes to people who are fasting for extended periods without making proper provisions regarding meals afterward, they may encounter the issue of overeating once their fast is broken, which could result in significant weight gain. To prevent this from occurring, people with diabetes engaging with intermittent fasting should plan out their meals beforehand that represent a combination of nutrients and low calories to keep any potential fluctuations in weight regulated during the course period. It must be taken into consideration, though, that while there can potentially be improved health outcomes associated with intermittent fasting, such as increased insulin sensitivity or enhanced cardiovascular performance, depending on how strictly one adheres to an IF regime based upon factors like current well-being status or pre-existing medical conditions like diabetes. Consequently, anyone considering implementing this lifestyle shift should consult a doctor. Hence, they have complete comprehension concerning all possible risks related to it before beginning anything at all.

Expert advice on Intermittent Fasting for diabetics

Intermittent fasting may be an attractive option for people with diabetes seeking to enhance their health. Instead of numerous diets highlighting calorie reduction, intermittent fasting focuses on managing when meals are consumed and how long people fast between mealtimes. By controlling the body's natural metabolic mechanisms, this approach could provide certain advantages over traditional dieting. Studies indicate that it might bring about advantageous metabolic transformations while permitting people with diabetes to meet their weight loss objectives without excluding entire food categories or drastically changing their diet plan.

For individuals with diabetes who are considering intermittent fasting, seeking professional advice before beginning any new dietary regimen is strongly recommended. The various potential benefits of such a practice for the alleviation or prevention of complications associated with diabetes, including heart disease and stroke due to improved blood sugar control as well as weight loss, have been examined by research around the world. Studies suggest this approach may help increase insulin sensitivity in type 1 and 2 diabetics.

Furthermore, many studies have proffered that periodic fasting could amplify physical prowess in individuals with type 1 diabetes because of increased insulin sensitivity. Nevertheless, it is imperative to comprehend that everyone's body chemistry differs - what works for one individual might not work for another - thus making it critically essential for people with diabetes to consult their physician before initiating any kind of new diet regimen, including intermittent fasting. Awareness of any potential pharmaceutical interactions or other medical complications connected with this system can facilitate assured success during someone's arranged fasts and eventually lead to better well-being in general.

Conclusion

Intermittent Fasting is a rising dietary trend that has demonstrated potential in regulating diabetes and its related symptoms. With a consistent fasting regimen, those affected by diabetes can benefit from keeping their blood glucose levels and controlling their body weight. Moreover, when the feeding window comes around, they should concentrate on whole foods so that nutrition-rich micronutrients will be prioritized along with overall diet quality. Intermit fasting should not substitute medical advice but must work together alongside professional healthcare guidance for optimal results.

Chapter 2:

Understanding Diabetes

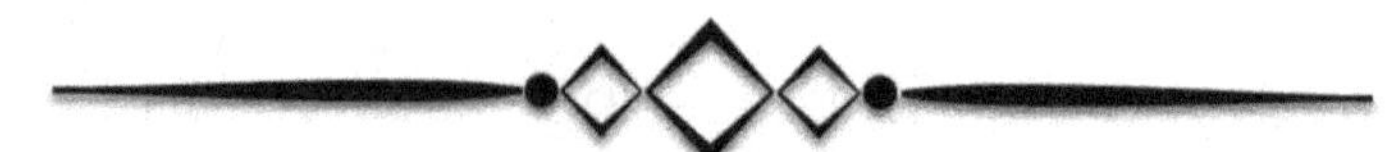

Are you affected by diabetes? It is a plight that affects millions of people around the world, and it can be complex to comprehend the principles of diabetes, monitor blood sugar levels, adhere to an appropriate diabetic diet, and learn how to manage this condition properly. This chapter assists in understanding the fundamentals of diabetes, its indicators, and manifestations, provides instruction on monitoring one's glucose concentrations, presents several recipes for nutritious diets appropriate for people with diabetes, and guides efficient ways to manage this illness.

What is the normal diabetes range?

It is essential to become aware of the conventional diabetic range. For people not diagnosed with diabetes, regular blood sugar (glucose) levels generally lie between 70 and 99 milligrams per deciliter (mg/dL). Blood glucose concentrations that exceed this norm may be an indication that prediabetes has occurred.

Prediabetes denotes when one's blood glucose levels surpass regular boundaries but have yet to reach the degree that would constitute a type 2 diabetes diagnosis. An A1C level between 5.7 and 6 can also be a marker for such circumstances.

Individuals with diabetes must maintain vigilance of their blood sugar levels and make lifestyle alterations, such as dietary differences or increased physical activity, to keep them at the target range. Regular consultations with medical professionals are necessary to monitor treatment progress and proactively manage any potential issues caused by this chronic illness. An A1C level below 4 percent suggests prediabetes, whereas anything over 6.5 percent indicates type 2 diabetes; however, these thresholds may vary depending on factors like age, activity level, and time of day. Those affected by type 1 diabetes whose bodies do not generate enough insulin to preserve optimal glucose concentrations in the bloodstream have a different reference value: readings higher than 130 mg/dL (in cases involving fasting) or 180 mg/dL (after meals) should be considered too high.

Common Symptoms Associated with Diabetes

Diabetes is a rapidly expanding health issue globally, so it is essential to recognize and accurately diagnose the condition. To do this, one must be aware of the common signs related to different forms of diabetes--Type 1 and Type 2--which can usually be divided into physical and metabolic manifestations. Biological indicators are often connected with high blood glucose levels, such as frequent urinating, intense thirstiness, and weight reduction without reasonable explanation, extreme hunger pangs, and weariness, changes in sight acuity, and wounds or cuts that heal slowly.

Metabolic issues may encompass nausea and vomiting, lightheadedness or dizziness when standing suddenly due to low blood sugar levels, and tingling sensations in the hands or feet caused by poor circulation. Notably, not all individuals with diabetes will experience these symptoms simultaneously - some might only present one or two. Nevertheless, if more than a single symptom persists for an extended time frame, it would be prudent to consult a doctor on the chance that diabetes should be excluded as its cause. Furthermore, prompt medical advice must be sought whenever sudden weight loss occurs without explanation since this could presumably indicate diabetes without other signs. By gaining familiarity with common manifestations connected to this disorder, people can recognize and address any potential difficulties before they become serious complications.

What are the four stages of diabetes?

It is widely acknowledged that Diabetes is a condition wherein the body cannot regulate its glucose levels, resulting in high blood sugar, and it has been observed to be on the rise among individuals from all age ranges around the globe. Therefore, it is critical to comprehend how this disease operates and what steps can be taken to manage it.

Generally speaking, there exist four stages of diabetes:

- ❖ Pre-diabetic state,
- ❖ Type 1 diabetes,
- ❖ Type 2 diabetes, and
- ❖ Gestational diabetes.

Pre-diabetics have their own particular set of symptoms where they exhibit higher than typical blood sugar levels, which may or might not meet the diagnosis criteria. At this stage, individuals do not necessarily require medication; they must make lifestyle modifications such as increasing exercise frequency or consuming a healthy diet. Those with prediabetes need to obtain regular testing to ascertain if their glucose levels have risen beyond the criteria for type 1 or type 2 diabetes.

Type 1 diabetes ensues when an individual's immune system attacks its cells responsible for insulin production, resulting in deficient amounts of insulin and ultimately increasing blood sugar levels.

In the case of people with type 1 diabetes, administering insulin injections and closely monitoring blood glucose levels are essential for maintaining good health.

Type 2 Diabetes is a state that arises when the body does not generate enough insulin, typically due to unhealthy lifestyle choices, including an inactive life paired with high-calorie diets resulting in obesity. It makes it more difficult for cells within the pancreas to produce sufficient levels of insulin essential for the proper functioning of the organism's cells, consequently leading to uncontrolled and elevated blood sugar levels. Similarly, as Type 1 Diabetic patients, those who have Type 2 Diabetes require daily injections of insulin or alternative medications alongside careful surveillance of their glucose intensity.

Gestational Diabetes is a condition that only affects pregnant women, typically disappearing after childbirth without any long-term health implications. Notwithstanding this, gestational diabetics have an increased chance of Type 2 Diabetes later in life. Thus, these individuals need to keep track of their glucose levels regularly and make the necessary adjustments to remain healthy. As one gets acquainted with each phase related to the disease, taking charge of personal healthcare becomes easier if falling within one or more categories associated with such conditions occurs. Proper management strategies such as dietary alterations and exercise plans tailored to individual requirements can enable persons to live healthier lives even when confronted with chronic ailments like diabetes.

Uncontrolled Blood Sugar: Implications and Risks

Uncontrolled blood sugar, or hyperglycemia, can have grave consequences for the well-being of an individual with diabetes. Even though dietary alterations and regular physical activity may help subside glucose levels in the bloodstream, there are situations where medication is required to maintain appropriate glycemic control. Research studies have demonstrated exposure over a long period to high blood sugar concentrations to cause harm or damage organs such as eyesight-related structures, kidneys, heart muscles, and peripheral nerves, essential elements within bodily systems. Additionally, it has been noted through examinations into this issue that uncontrolled diabetes increases mortality rates due to complications resulting from cardiovascular diseases.

The factors contributing to hyperglycemia are manifold, comprising lifestyle decisions such as a poor diet, lack of physical activity, and genetic components. Moreover, certain medications can also cause an increase in blood glucose levels. Persons with diabetes experience heightened vulnerability during times of illness or stress due to the body's natural generation of hormones like cortisol that momentarily boost the requirement for energy; this may lead to surges in insulin resistance and ensuing high amounts of glucose if it is not appropriately managed through changes comprised within one's dietary regime or other interventions.

The effective maintenance of Diabetes is a fundamental factor for long-term health outcomes. It must be customized to each person's unique requirements based on their medical background, lifestyle choices, family support structure, and access to healthcare services. Regular consultations with a primary care provider can advise how best to keep track of glucose levels in the long run while also handling accompanying conditions that might make it challenging to maintain glycemic control, such as hypertension or cholesterol irregularities. Moreover, most states offer free programs like authorized diabetes education courses, which provide thorough training on building balanced meal plans and direction concerning adherence to medication if necessary.

Understanding the Diabetes Diet: Foods to Include

People with type 2 diabetes must maintain a low saturated fats and high-fiber diet. Specifically, such diets should reduce sugar and carbohydrates while incorporating non-starchy vegetables, lean proteins, fiber-rich whole grains, and heart-healthy fats to provide essential vitamins and minerals while maintaining stable blood sugar levels.

Vegetables such as spinach, kale, broccoli, and carrots are all sensible selections for dietary inclusion. Furthermore, consuming a variety of colors may ensure that individuals obtain the complete spectrum of vitamins and minerals they require nutritionally. Lean proteins should be incorporated into diets to regulate diabetes, guaranteeing the body receives adequate protein while avoiding excessive saturated fat or calories. Eggs, fish, poultry products, beans, and nuts constitute exemplary sources of lean proteins; ingesting several servings facilitates essential amino acids without excessively augmenting fat or caloric levels within meals.

Including a variety of fiber-rich whole grains in the diet is essential for individuals with diabetes, as they provide essential nutrients and help to regulate blood sugar levels. Examples of suitable choices include oats, barley, quinoa, and brown rice; these can be consumed regularly throughout the day as part of meals or snacks. Moreover, heart-healthy fats should also form an essential component of this dietary plan. Still, it is vital to remember that moderation must be practiced when selecting such foods so saturated fat intake does not become excessive or calories overly abundant. Olive oil represents one great choice within this category, along with avocados and nuts like almonds or walnuts, which render dishes more appetizing while encouraging optimal health conditions by managing blood sugars effectively.

Foods to Avoid in a Diabetes Diet

Comprehending diabetes and managing it through diet is crucial to successfully regulating it. Knowing which foods should be disregarded and why they must not be consumed is essential to retain wholesome blood sugar levels. Below are some primarily significant kinds of food that an individual with diabetes should avoid or at least restrict their ingestion to keep their glucose level within the desired range. Refined carbohydrates, including white rice, white bread, and sugary snacks, are all high glycemic index (GI) foods that should be avoided in the context of a diabetes-friendly diet. Such items can rapidly elevate blood sugar levels within the body, resulting in fluctuations that harm health if experienced consistently over an extended period. It is recommended to consume lower GI grains such as brown rice, oats, and quinoa instead. In addition to this, processed meats should also not be consumed when attempting to manage diabetes through dietary means.

Many processed meats such as sausages, bacon, and salami have large quantities of carbohydrates and drenched fat, which causes weight gain if they are consumed too frequently. A better option would be lean proteins like egg whites, grilled chicken, or fish that do not contain additional sugars and possess much less saturated fat than processed meats.

In addition, those with diabetes must restrict their intake of full-fat dairy products, including cheese, cream, or yogurt, as these options are high in calories yet simple to accumulate into substantial amounts without being mindful about eating habits. Low-fat varieties tend to be substantially lower in calorific content while providing similar nutrient benefits to other dairy items. Thus, they often work as a healthier substitute for people with diabetes who wish for an occasional indulgence but refrain from exceeding their calorie consumption limits.

Steps towards Effective Diabetes Management

Accurate diagnosis of diabetes is the 1st step in successful management. It typically necessitates performing various tests, including blood and glucose tolerance tests, to pinpoint whether an individual has diabetes. Subsequently, it is critical to monitor glucose levels closely using one or both approaches - regular lab testing or a daily at-home monitoring system for greater control over fluctuations in blood sugar levels that can be harmful if not detected quickly enough.

Patients are encouraged to make healthy lifestyle changes to manage their diabetes better. Adopting a balanced diet with regular meals that reduce sugary food intake can be instrumental in effectively managing the condition. Furthermore, engaging regularly in physical activity aids the maintenance of ideal insulin levels while promoting general well-being.

If dietary modifications and exercise alone do not suffice, medication may become necessary to keep glucose levels under control; this typically involves either specific types of oral or injectable drugs taken daily or periodically as prescribed by a doctor who will provide clear instructions regarding dosage based on readings from blood sugar testing throughout the day alongside pre-meal reminders if applicable.

Moreover, people living with diabetes need to pay close attention to any other conditions that could affect its management over time, such as high cholesterol or hypertension caused by unhealthy practices like smoking and drinking alcohol excessively; keeping track of these afflictions contributes to achieving successful long-term management goals associated with leading a healthy life free from complications arising out of having diabetes.

How do you know if you have type 1 or 2 diabetes?

It is paramount to distinguish between Type 1 and Type 2 diabetes to decide the optimal course of action for managing the condition.

Type 1 diabetes appears when the pancreas produces negligible or no insulin, a hormone that allows the body to use glucose from food as energy. This form of diabetes generally appears during childhood or early adolescence and necessitates continual treatment with insulin injections.

In contrast to Type 1 diabetes, which transpires when the body does not produce insulin at all, Type 2 diabetes is a condition in which either an insufficient amount of insulin is made, or it cannot be utilized correctly by the body, resulting in elevated glucose levels within one's bloodstream. Generally occurring during adulthood, this disorder can also manifest itself among children; its onset has been associated with family history and being overweight.

To determine whether an individual has type 1 or type 2 diabetes, a medical professional may perform tests such as measuring the amount of glucose in one's bloodstream at various points throughout the day, evaluating if their body is releasing sufficient insulin, examining if cells can respond correctly to insulin; and assessing if sugar metabolism is overactive which could be indicative of poor cell response towards insulin. Furthermore, signs like weight loss and intense thirst can hint towards having type 1 diabetes. After performing these tests, a doctor will make a confirmatory diagnosis depending on test results, symptoms present, and any family history associated with this condition.

What stage of diabetes is severe?

Diabetes is a severe metabolic ailment that affects millions of people globally. Regarding diabetes, it is essential to comprehend that there are various stages of the sickness, including prediabetes, type 1 diabetes, and kind two diabetes. Of all these phases, which set of diabetes is serious? Type 1 and type 2 Diabetes are the two most prevalent types of this illness and can be exceedingly intense if not attended to or appropriately controlled. Type 1 Diabetes is an autoimmune condition in which the pancreas produces little Insulin.

Individuals with Type 1 Diabetes must maintain their blood sugar levels within a specific range via regular insulin injections to avoid potentially life-threatening consequences such as heart attack, stroke, renal defeat, and blindness. Therefore, individuals suffering from this condition should take the necessary steps to vigilantly monitor their glucose levels while properly administering suitable insulin doses when needed. On the other hand, Type 2 Diabetes is generally known as either Adult Onset or Lifestyle Related Diabetes.

In the case of Type 2 Diabetes, a lack of sufficient insulin production or cellular resistance to its effects results in elevated blood sugar levels. If not managed appropriately, individuals living with this form of Diabetes are at risk for severe consequences like heart attack, nerve damage, organ failure, and even death. Proper management requires lifestyle adjustments such as lowering intake from sources including processed food products and sugary drinks while increasing consumption from whole-grain foods such as quinoa and brown rice; exercise is also an essential element in any successful care plan. All told both types 1 and 2 Diabetes can be severe if left unaddressed or uncontrolled due to their potential long-term health outcomes, including mortality in some cases when no management efforts have been taken up.

Exercise and Lifestyle Changes for Diabetes Control

Those managing diabetes must engage in regular exercise and lifestyle changes, which can help reduce and maintain healthy blood sugar levels. Exercise has been proven to regulate insulin resistance, decrease cardiovascular risks, enhance overall health, increase energy levels, and bolster confidence. Additionally, making dietary modifications such as limiting alcohol consumption, quitting smoking, and ensuring adequate restful sleep are also essential components of controlling diabetes. It would be wise for an individual with diabetes to speak with a dietitian or nutritionist so that they may develop personalized diets based on their own needs. It should consist of complex carbohydrates paired with proteins while incorporating unsaturated fats over saturated ones; additionally, keeping meals relatively low-fat while including plenty of fresh fruits & vegetables is another significant factor when cultivating nourishing eating habits. Continuing down the path towards poorly managed diabetes could lead to further complications that affect various organs within the body; thus, it stands paramount that people living day by day who are diagnosed with Type 1 or 2 Diabetes must ensure their respective exercise regimes stay up-to-date alongside maintaining balanced diets -allowing them tremendous success concerning long term management efforts relating all around to one's diagnosis.

Conclusion

It is imperative to comprehend diabetes to gain control over this condition and avoid any future health problems. Through education about its fundamentals, signs, and symptoms, as well as management methods related to diabetes, individuals can make prudent lifestyle decisions that advocate a balanced diet alongside other techniques to uphold normality regarding their blood sugar levels. By preserving these points in mind, people can maximize their quality of life while better-regulating diabetes.

Chapter 3:

Intermittent Fasting Basics

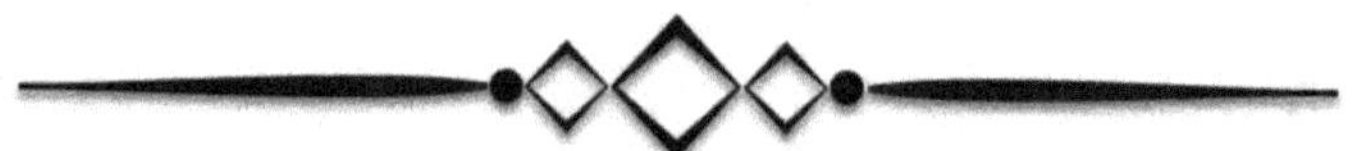

Intermittent Fasting is gaining prominence as a valuable element of well-being, particularly for those with diabetes. Intermittent Fasting consists of periods of eating and fasting that help the body burn fat, regulate blood sugar levels, and maintain an optimal weight. The fundamentals associated with intermittent fasting are its advantages in managing diabetes diets while ensuring healthy dietary habits. Consequently, if you are eager to learn more about intermittent fasting or plan to commence this practice, please read further to understand all foundational aspects and rewards relevant to individuals affected by diabetes.

What is the fasting goal for people with diabetes?

Adopting an intermittent fasting diet can be advantageous for individuals with diabetes, yet it is imperative to comprehend why and how this eating regimen works. Intermittent fasting includes expanding during specific occasions of the day while declining from nourishment amid different circumstances. The reason for this training regularly centers around keeping up consistent blood glucose levels. For those battling type 2 diabetes, monitoring glucose dimensions is essential to keep side effects in line.

Fasting is beneficial for individuals who are overweight or obese and has been interpreted with type 2 diabetes, as it assists in weight control. Furthermore, when choosing carbohydrate-rich foods that meet the fasting goal for diabetics, two primary goals should be kept in mind: timing and content. Choosing complex carbohydrates such as whole grains, legumes, and vegetables is preferable over highly processed sources like white bread; quality matters more than quantity regarding managing blood sugar levels. Additionally, taking into account the time of day at which these carbohydrates are consumed can help reduce fluctuations of blood glucose levels; research shows that eating a combination of healthy fat along with protein and complex carbs somewhat earlier on during the day helps improve glycemic control compared with having most of the said carbs later up until nightfall.

Detailed Explanation of Fasting Basics

Intermittent fasting has recently gained much attention as a productive method for achieving health and weight loss results. Incorporating fasting into one's lifestyle is uncomplicated, providing valuable advantages to those struggling with diabetes. Recognizing how intermittent fasting works is essential to obtain the best outcomes from this practice. Fundamentals of intermittent fasting are indispensable for any person desirous of using intermittent fasting safely and effectively. Fasting encompasses abstaining from food or drink, typically during a predetermined time interval between 12 to 72 hours.

Throughout this period, no calories are ingested, and the body employs stored energy (generally fat) as a power source. This action affords the digestive system an urgently needed respite, permitting the physique to reset and rejuvenate itself before eating again. Additionally, it assists in stabilizing insulin levels by diminishing tension in one's pancreas and providing time for recovery between meals. For those struggling with diabetes, intermittent fasting can be advantageous in many ways, such as lessening inflammatory biomarkers in their blood, which may lead to increased insulin sensitivity.

By keeping meals regular but spaced farther apart, one may enjoy fewer spikes in blood sugar levels throughout the day, which can assist in reducing the overall risk of cardiovascular issues related to diabetes, such as stroke and hypertension. Moreover, intermittent fasting facilitates healthy weight loss with a proper exercise routine. It does not need to be done every day; two or three times per week is sufficient for reaping its benefits. When engaging in this practice, individuals must remain well-hydrated since dehydration could significantly alter their blood sugar levels, resulting in further complications concerning diabetes management. Additionally, during fasting intervals, it is essential to listen closely to one's body; if extreme fatigue or dizziness is experienced, eating something light before continuing would be recommended.

How to control diabetes with fasting?

Fasting has become a well-known technique of dietary intervention for people with diabetes. This practice can be conducted on either an intermittent or constant basis, depending upon the specific requirements and preferences of each individual. Intermittent fasting involves alternating periods involving consumption and abstention from eating. Even though it is rapidly gaining traction recently, fasting cannot be considered a new concept as it has been employed extensively over numerous years to treat several ailments such as diabetes. Research findings have demonstrated that intermittent fasting may benefit metabolic health in those with type 2 diabetes; this incorporates augmented insulin sensitivity, decreased inflammation, and optimized glucose regulation. Fasting has the additional benefit of reducing body fat and promoting weight loss, which can help manage diabetes-related complications such as hypertension and cardiovascular disease. To control blood sugar levels during fasting periods effectively, individuals should take preventive measures like monitoring glucose levels vigilantly and ensuring proper hydration with noncaloric liquids, including water or herbal tea. Additionally, ingesting low-carbohydrate meals before a fast may sustain evenness of blood sugar concentrations throughout the duration that one abstains from food intake. Finally, given that intermittent fasting could potentially lead to decreased appetite levels and energy expenditure at certain times, it is essential for people who practice this dietary regimen to make sure they are getting adequate rest and nourishment over their non-fasting hours for overall good health plus prudent regulation of bloodstream glucose measurements.

What type of intermittent fasting is best for prediabetes?

Intermittent fasting is a popular dietary strategy connected to various health advantages, including the potential to decrease the dangers of developing prediabetes. Nevertheless, it is critical to comprehend which type of intermittent fasting might be most appropriate for those potentially suffering from prediabetes. Although there are multiple versions of this method of consuming foodstuffs, they can usually be classified into two large groups: daily time-restricted diets and periodic abstinence from nourishment. Daily time-restricted diets necessitate diminishing consumption during specific periods or days each week.

Regarding people predisposed to diabetes, recent studies suggest that a combination of daily time-restricted diets and periodic fasts may most effectively reduce its associated risk. Considering individual circumstances, an appropriate amount or type of intermittent fasting should be discussed with a medical professional before initiating any new diet plan. Additionally, research indicates that daily time-restricted diets have the potential to regulate blood sugar levels while offering extra energy due to shortened periods between meals; furthermore, prolonged periods without food through periodic fasts can diminish inflammation within the body, which could lead pre-diabetic conditions such as insulin resistance and excessive fat gain.

Exploring the Benefits of Intermittent Fasting for Diabetes

Intermittent fasting garners expanded notice in the governance of diabetes and its accompanying symptoms. Although additional research is necessary to discover the complete potentiality of this kind of dietary intervention, early outcomes demonstrate possibilities for those with diabetes. Intermittent fasting has been observed to enhance glycemic control, diminish human fat, and strengthen insulin sensitivity among individuals with type 2 diabetes. Added evidence implies that intermittent fasting could also decrease blood pressure and cholesterol levels in persons diagnosed with diabetes.

Furthermore, intermittent fasting may ameliorate overall energy levels by bolstering and maintaining glucose concentrations within the body. These discoveries are encouraging news for those with diabetes who aspire to stay energetic and healthful in their later years. Consequently, people with diabetes should focus on consuming various nutrient-dense foods such as fruits, vegetables, whole grains, lean proteins, and healthy fats.

Eliminating processed or refined carbohydrates is essential to preserve optimal blood sugar levels and hinder undesired weight gain, which can further exacerbate many diabetic complications. In addition, the incorporation of intermittent fasting practices into one's diet may give even more advantages for those living with diabetes who are seeking to manage their condition more effectively.

There are various methods of intermittent fasting to choose from, such as the 5:2 diet or alternate-day fasting, based on individual needs and preferences. Said practices generally involve periods where food is limited, followed by times when it can be eaten commonly. During periods of restriction, it is essential to intake enough water; however, consuming other beverages should only occur if guided by a physician or nutritionist. Additionally, for those taking prescription drugs for diabetes conditions, consulting with a healthcare practitioner before modifying their lifestyle routine is recommended.

Healthy Eating Habits to Compliment Intermittent Fasting

It is essential that individuals who are engaged in intermittent fasting and those desiring to better their health maintain healthy eating habits. Eating nutrient-rich foods and abstaining from processed food may assist with attaining superior well-being results. About intermittent fasting, which consists of an often-used pattern wherein periods of abstinence from consuming alternate with times of ingestion, it is essential to center on whole foods, which can help meet the body's necessities. Foods naturally that contain many nutrients, antioxidants, fiber, and protein can aid in regulating blood sugar levels while providing sustained energy levels.

Intermittent fasting can be significantly supplemented by eating plenty of plant-based proteins such as legumes and nuts. Add healthy fats, including avocados, olive oil, or coconut oil, and it is also advisable to remain satiated throughout the fast. Additionally, one's well-being needs to stay hydrated with water rather than juices or sugary drinks during this period. Furthermore, packaged snacks should be avoided whenever possible since they are often high in carbohydrates and sugar, which could lead to spikes in blood glucose levels if overconsumed regularly. Adding these nutritional habits into one's lifestyle while intermittently fasting may improve mental clarity and sleep patterns, thus significantly improving overall wellness.

The Link between Diabetes Diet and Intermittent Fasting

Regarding diabetes, diet, and nutrition are of the utmost importance. Recently, intermittent fasting has been one of the more well-known dietary trends to have gathered intensity. Although conceptually, fasting is not an entirely novel notion, comprehending how it pertains to diabetes might benefit those pursuing lifestyle changes. Intermittent fasting involves periods alternating between eating and fasting, which can significantly influence blood sugar levels and overall health.

Regarding the association between diabetes and intermittent fasting, multiple advantages can be attained with the correct execution of this kind of diet. Studies have demonstrated that when combined with a wholesome diet and exercise program, intermittent fasting can enhance glycemic control for those with Type 2 diabetes. Consequently, blood sugar levels remain consistent throughout the day, reducing both rises and drops in glucose concentrations.

Studies have demonstrated that Intermittent Fasting (IF) is an effective way of aiding weight loss and sustaining a healthy body mass over time because it minimizes caloric intake without making individuals experience undue deprivation or hunger. Moreover, incorporating intermittent fasting into the diet plan of somebody with diabetes has been seen to reduce cholesterol levels while maintaining healthy blood pressure readings. A recent study analyzed two dietary programs for people with Type 2 Diabetes - an IFD combined with a continuous energy restriction scheme (CER)- observed across six-month durations.

The results demonstrated that, compared to the control group following a CER protocol, those individuals adhering to an IFD regimen exhibited improved lipid profiles due to increased fat loss. Incorporating intermittent fasting into a diabetic lifestyle may assist in reducing inflammation through various mechanisms, such as diminishing pro-inflammatory cytokines and augmenting anti-inflammatory proteins within the body; this could lead to decreased risk for long-term diseases like cardiovascular disease or strokeover time. Considering its potential advantages, healthcare professionals should provide Type 2 Diabetes patients with education about Intermittent Fasting as part of their comprehensive diet plan along with traditional methods, including counting carbohydrate intake and monitoring glucose levels regularly.

How Intermittent Fasting Affects Your Blood Sugar Levels

Intermittent Fasting is a widely utilized dietary technique that has the potential to aid in the management of blood glucose levels, particularly for those with Type 2 diabetes. During periods of intermittent fasting, no nourishment is consumed by the body within a designated timeframe, which assists in the augmentation of one's native capacity to synthesize insulin, manage sugar concentrations, and reduce inflammation.

Moreover, intermittent fasting may also assist in mitigating risks related to the evolution of Type 2 Diabetes by contributing towards weight reduction and surging metabolism involving sugars. Regarding the regulation of blood glucose levels, intermittent fasting can be advantageous.

Providing the body with an opportunity to fast allows for burning off any surplus glycogen stores and increased sensitivity towards insulin. It subsequently enables a more efficient breakdown of carbohydrates consumed during meals, thus reducing post-meal glucose levels. As prolonged high blood sugar will raise one's chances of suffering from diabetes complications such as nerve damage and kidney disease, it is essential for people with diabetes who opt to fast to keep their post-meal glucose spikes low.

A recent study found that eighteen to twenty-four-hour fasting periods over eight weeks significantly impacted glucose uptake and insulin resistance in obese patients with type 2 diabetes.[1] Another investigation carried out among non-diabetic adults demonstrated the efficacy of intermittent fasting for improved glycemic control overall.[2] Consequently, people with diabetes may be able to better manage their blood sugar levels through the regular practice of this dietary restriction – whether by abstaining from breakfast or partaking in alternate-day fasts.

Moreover, numerous other health benefits have been associated with systematic intermittent fasting, such as enhanced digestion, cognitive function, and cardiovascular health, which is why it has recently become popular.[3] However, caution must be taken since those individuals who have type 2 diabetes should consider how periodic lengthy fasts will affect absorption rate when taking medication as well as caloric needs before making any long-lasting decisions,[4] but if done correctly, can offer advantages to managing their condition more effectively.

Tips for Starting and Maintaining Intermittent Fasting for Diabetes

Intermittent fasting can be a possible option for managing diabetes due to its capacity to provide advantages such as weight loss and the decreased chance of mourning from stroke or heart attack. When executed correctly, intermittent fasting may also reduce blood sugar levels and help control hormones in diabetic individuals. It is essential to observe one's body signals while initiating it gently. The following advice should prove beneficial when starting with an intermitted festive program for those who have diabetes:

It is imperative to seek the advice of a doctor before initiating an intermittent fasting regime, particularly for those living with diabetes. A physician must confirm if this dietary practice is secure for someone with diabetes. Furthermore, it is crucial that any eating plan adopted by persons affected with diabetes does not conflict with any medications being taken and that they routinely monitor their blood sugar levels at commencement to guarantee its successful operation.

Additionally, there are various forms of intermittent fasting available. For those with type

2 diabetes, it may be advantageous to initiate their exploration into this method of nourishment by commencing a 12-hour fast followed by twelve hours, wherein food is permitted every 24 hours. Only calorie-free drinks such as water or herbal teas should be ingested during the fasting interval. After becoming accustomed to this pattern on behalf of the body, other variants like 16/8 can be attempted if desired.

Thirdly, due to the potential impacts intermittent fasting may have on individuals living with diabetes in terms of their blood glucose levels, it is advisable for those commencing this lifestyle change to gradually reintroduce carbohydrates after meals once they become accustomed to consuming meals during predetermined eating windows each day. It will give people sufficient time between meal times, enabling them to keep track and respond promptly if a rise in sugar level occurs while transitioning from fasts into feasts or vice versa.

Ultimately, developing mindful eating habits in combination with intermittent fasting can help promote better dietary choices while managing diabetes overall. These behaviors include heightening awareness of hunger signals before consuming meals or snacks, spacing out consumption throughout the day instead of binging on huge portions at a time since people who do this tend to eat more than if they had smaller amounts over designated periods during their fasts and paying attention to fullness cues after having eaten rather than continuing until feeling content or "full" while living life within an intermittent fasting schedule as well as concurrently managing type 2 diabetes.

Conclusion

Intermittent fasting has proven to be an advantageous and practical approach to managing diabetes. Not only does it aid in improving blood sugar control and reducing inflammation, but it also promotes the development of healthier eating habits. Those considering engaging with this form of practice must gain a basic understanding of meal timing and follow a healthy diet; furthermore, consultation with one's healthcare provider should occur so they can craft an individualized plan tailor-made specifically for them. By making some minor changes alongside dedication towards following through on their routine, individuals have the potential to

revolutionize how they manage their diabetes by
utilizing intermittent fasting methods effectively.

Chapter 4:

The Science Behind Intermittent Fasting and Blood Sugar

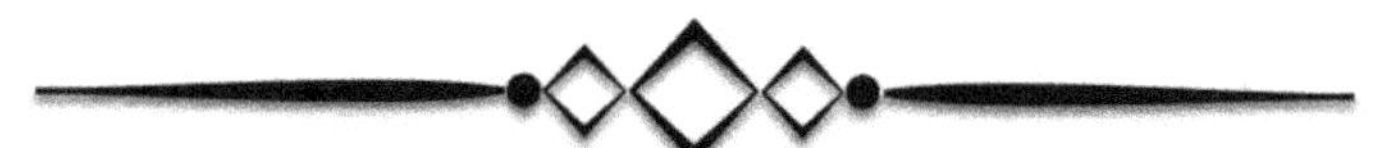

Intermittent fasting has become famous for its potential health benefits, but some are concerned about its impact on glucose levels. This text investigates the scientific fundamentals regarding intermittent fasting and explores how it affects your body's glucose measurement. We will consider both advantages and dangers when considering adopting an abstaining diet plan and analyzing research that elucidates such decisions, allowing one to make an educated conclusion.

Importance of Blood Sugar Regulation

Regulation of blood sugar is an essential part of the human body and must be kept in a proportionate range to ensure proper functioning. Intermittent fasting (IF) has become quite popular as an approach for controlling glucose levels, as it can aid with reducing insulin resistance, enhancing glucose metabolism, and minimizing general caloric intake. For instance, IF may reduce appetite and cravings for hazardous foods or snacks, which could result in improved adherence to a low-calorie diet plan. Additionally, research studies have demonstrated that IF might also lessen inflammation caused by high-fat meals, consequently having potential healing effects in preventing metabolic disorders such as diabetes mellitus and obesity. Moreover, IF will assist with prohibiting muscle loss during dieting since it facilitates the preservation of muscle mass yet encourages the body to utilize fat deposits instead for energy production. Intermittent fasting should be incorporated into healthy lifestyle choices and other approaches to regulate blood sugar, including regular physical exercise routine and mindful eating habits."

Understanding Insulin Sensitivity

The body's capacity to be attentive to the impacts of insulin is a fundamental factor in health and wellness. When individuals have sound insulin sensitivity, their bodies can more effectively convert the energy produced from food into helpful fuel for their cells. It explains why recognizing insulin sensitivity is advantageous for maintaining blood sugar levels. With suitable glucose control, one can guarantee they remain vigorous and active regularly.

Furthermore, having good insulin sensitivity allows individuals to more competently process carbohydrates without facing too high an increase in blood sugar levels. Consequently, learning about how insulin sensitivity works can assist people with getting the most out of their diet and lifestyle decisions to realize optimal health and well-being. Notably, those who pursue intermittent fasting are likely to observe an enhancement in their insulin sensitivity due to giving the body intermissions between meals containing tiny amounts of sugar. Additionally, supplementing with herbs such as berberine is believed to aid progress towards improved glucose consumption for those struggling with Type 2 Diabetes or other conditions related to overconsumption of sugar. Therefore, comprehending how insulin operates inside someone's body proves vital when striving for overall well-being and equilibrium concerning one's physical condition.

How Intermittent Fasting Affects Insulin Sensitivity

Intermittent Fasting, also comprehended as time-restricted eating, has recently become popular among those concerned with health and wellness. This dietary approach limits food consumption to specific times during the day. While research exists regarding its probable benefits on overall health, studies into how it impacts insulin sensitivity are still in their infancy; however, what is available does point towards improved glucose tolerance and decreased risk for any diabetes-associated conditions. A survey revealed that intermittent fasting reduced basal and postprandial insulin levels amongst overweight subjects with type 2 diabetes.

The researchers concluded that regular fasting periods could reduce insulin resistance and enhance overall glycemic control for individuals with this condition. Moreover, another study determined that alternate-day fasting caused nearly a 60% reduction in plasma insulin concentrations compared to the continuous caloric restriction group, thus bolstering the notion that intermittent fasting positively affects insulin sensitivity.

Likewise, animal studies have provided added evidence concerning how intermittent fasting may affect glucose metabolism. For instance, periodic fasts were discovered to better key metabolic markers associated with type 2 diabetes, such as triglyceride levels and muscle glycogen content. Additionally, these fasts resulted in lower circulating amounts of leptin and ghrelin hormones, which are responsible for appetite control regulation and food intake, respectively.

Overall, it can be seen from all findings that carrying out occasional intervals of abstinence over an extensive period appears to lead positively toward improving insulin sensitivity and glucose homeostasis within sufferers. Such beneficial outcomes might prove advantageous, particularly for those who risk developing diabetes or managing its medical implications accordingly.

Effects of Intermittent Fasting on Body's Glucose Levels

In recent years, Intermittent Fasting (IF) has become increasingly widespread due to its potential health benefits, chief among them being its beneficial influence on blood sugar levels. Studies suggest that IF can regulate glucose concentrations and reduce one's risk of developing type 2 diabetes by altering hormones released in the body, enabling greater control over the production and release of glucose. People who practice IF are likely to maintain lower average blood sugar values than those who do not, as fasting allows more efficient storage of stored energy to prevent sudden spikes in glycemia. Additionally, intermittent fasting may improve insulin sensitivity, thereby making it easier for cells to absorb available sugars from ingested food sources while also increasing GLP-1 production, a hormone known to normalize blood sugar levels, thus reducing an individual's exposure or vulnerability concerning developing diabetic conditions or related complications associated in addition to that can be minimized through intermittent fasting techniques applied frequently at suitable intervals.

Research and Studies on Intermittent Fasting and Insulin Sensitivity

An increasing body of research has been done to consider the impact of intermittent fasting on insulin sensitivity. Intermittent fasting is an eating method that cycles between times when calorie consumption is limited and regular food intake occurs. Studies have found that during durations of intermittent fasting, production by the body of insulin diminishes. Insulin plays a significant role in keeping blood glucose levels steady as it aids cells in taking up glucose from circulation within the bloodstream. Lowering amounts of insulin can result in improved metabolic health outcomes and cheaper rates of blood sugar levels. Moreover, studies also present evidence suggesting increased generation using intermittent fasting associated with adiponectin - a hormone connected with enhanced senses towards insulin plus better metabolism overall; additionally, investigators have discovered fastings mediate autophagy, which involves the breakdown organized by cells so damaged or unneeded proteins alongside organelles are recycled or eliminated promoting lessened inflammation inside bodies thus improving awareness regarding insulins furthermore all together improving general metabolic wellness through interim fastings."

Reducing Insulin Resistance through Intermittent Fasting

Physical activity and dietary alterations constitute the most vital aspects of a lifestyle conducive to reducing insulin resistance. Intermittent fasting has been attested as one such approach that can be beneficial in controlling insulin resistance and keeping glucose levels healthy. Recent research studies have demonstrated that intermittent fasting may ameliorate glucose metabolism and lower blood sugar concentration among persons with type 2 diabetes or prediabetes conditions. Interval fasting encompasses restricting caloric intake over concise periods, usually from 16 to 24 hours.

During these periods of fasting, the body will access its fat stores for energy instead of relying on glucose from the food consumed in prior meals. This mechanism increases metabolic flexibility and reduces insulin resistance by lowering the amount of glucose released into circulation at any moment. Moreover, research has demonstrated that intermittent fasting can boost adiponectin production, a hormone linked with increased insulin sensitivity and superior control over blood sugar levels.

Approaching intermittent fasting should be done since it is not appropriate for everyone; those with hypoglycemia or other medical conditions may need to adjust their routine accordingly. It is recommended to converse with one's doctor before starting up an intermittent fast regimen, especially if you are taking medications or have a health issue that changes or restrictions in dietary habits could impact.

Balancing Blood Sugar Levels with Intermittent Fasting

The practice of intermittent fasting has received escalated focus in the last few years due to its potential health benefits. Studies demonstrate that it can aid weight loss, enhance metabolic well-being, and lessen inflammation. Moreover, some investigations suggest it may help balance blood glucose concentrations. This essay will investigate the science behind intermittent fasting and how this impacts our levels of blood sugar.

It is critical to comprehend what transpires when we consume meals.

Upon consumption of carbohydrates, they are broken down into glucose, which is then absorbed by the bloodstream and utilized for energy. It triggers a heightened release of insulin from the pancreas to transport the glucose out of the blood and into cells, which can be used as fuel or stored away for future use. Suppose an excessive quantity of insulin has been released or cells have become resistant to this hormone. In that case, elevated glucose levels remain in the bloodstream, thus resulting in high blood sugar (hyperglycemia).

Intermittent fasting influences this process due to lowered meal frequency, thus resulting in a diminished intake of carbohydrates altogether. It consequently leads to a smaller quantity of glucose entering the bloodstream, reducing insulin secretion stimulation from the pancreas.

With less glucose present, cells need no more energy, which causes them to take up further amounts of glucose released into circulation; this is beneficial in restoring high blood sugar levels to their typical range.

As the frequency of meals decreases over time, our body's ability to respond appropriately to insulin decreases as well; this is an advantageous result when considering balancing our blood sugar levels. Additionally, research conducted on animals indicates that intermittent fasting can lead to increased glucagon production, which helps manage energy pathways by enabling stored energy (glucose) from liver cells in circulation, offsetting rising glycemic readings, particularly during times when food intake or caloric restriction takes place, such as through the night hours and successive periods between meals while following periodic fasts protocols. Moreover, recent investigations reveal that if one combines intermittent fasting with changes in dieting habits, for example, decreased consumption and consistent exercising, more significant effects could be achieved toward sustaining healthy blood glucose compared to utilizing either way exclusively - thus indicating its possible role concerning controlling hyperglycemia correlated matters like diabetes type II regulation.

Practical Tips for Implementing Intermittent Fasting for Blood Sugar Control

Studies have shown intermittent fasting can be an emphatic tool to regulate blood sugar levels. It has been demonstrated that engaging in periods of fasting leads to increased insulin sensitivity, decreased fat content, and improved overall health and quality of life. Nevertheless, one must understand the scientific principles behind this method to maximize its effects on controlling blood sugar levels.

The fundamental concept surrounding intermittent fasting involves:

- Reducing carbohydrate intake while increasing dietary fats.

- Essentially, eating fewer carbohydrates than what would typically be consumed throughout the day.

- Avoiding snacks between meals or post-dinner timeframes altogether.

By diminishing the quantity of carbohydrates ingested, the body enters a state of ketosis, which assists in burning fat more productively for energy generation rather than carbohydrates. Consequently, this aids in decreasing circulating glucose concentrations within the bloodstream, ultimately facilitating improved blood sugar control after some time. Another pragmatic hint towards enforcing intermittent fasting for controlling one's glucose level involves consuming healthy fats such as olive oil, coconut oil, avocados, and nuts throughout the day instead of overconsuming carbohydrate intake.

Healthy fats can be beneficial in stabilizing blood glucose levels, as they slow digestion and provide sustained energy over a more extended period, contrasted with carbohydrates, which often cause spikes in glucose concentrations. Furthermore, consuming high-fiber foods such as legumes, vegetables, and whole grains may be advantageous for controlling blood sugar levels due to providing essential vitamins and minerals that help optimize metabolism, eventually leading to improved glucose tolerance. Finally, it is also critical to maintain balance between these elements by taking adequate amounts of protein throughout the day because proteins inherently affect glucose stabilization owing to their slower rate of digestion than those associated with either carbohydrates or fats.

Personalized Approaches to Blood Sugar Management

A personalized approach to blood sugar management has the potential to make a buoyant contribution towards an individual's health and well-being. The intricacy of the physiologic and metabolic processes in regulating blood sugar levels makes it complex to formulate a single diet or exercise routine conducive to optimal wellness. A plan that may be effective for one person might not necessarily bring about favorable results concerning another, and vice versa; this is why designing tailored programs considering each person's exceptional metabolism and lifestyle can aid them in controlling their glucose concentrations.

When it comes to personalized approaches for blood sugar management, careful consideration is required of food intake, physical activity, medications, and the influence that stress levels, sleep habits, and other factors can have on glycemic control. One dietary strategy increasingly used to regulate these parameters is intermittent fasting, which involves consuming all meals within a certain number of hours each day or abstaining from food entirely during specific periods. Advocates suggest this system helps manage hormones connected with hunger and satiety while activating metabolic pathways beneficial for healthy glucose regulation. However, intermittent fasting may not always be appropriate or safe; hence, individuals with diabetes should contact their healthcare provider before committing to such regimes.

Conclusion

Intermittent Fasting is a highly effective method of managing blood sugar and insulin levels. The science behind it can be trusted to provide accurate results, and the benefits are plentiful. Research has indicated that this form of fasting may decrease glucose concentrations in healthy people and those with diabetes by increasing insulin sensitivity while aiding metabolic health overall. As has always been stressed, if one wishes to initiate any dietary regime or alterations in lifestyle habits, they should seek consultation from their physician first to ensure it suits their needs.

Chapter 5:

Preparing to Start Intermittent Fasting

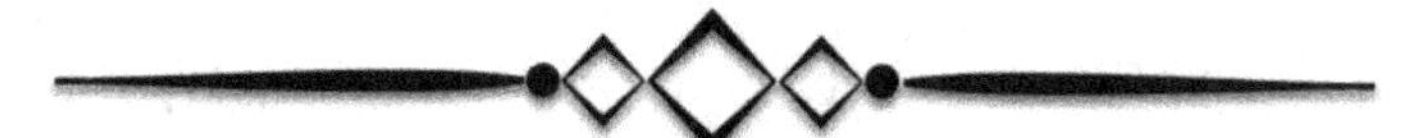

Diabetic Patients considering the lifestyle of intermittent fasting should be aware of its influence on their diabetes management and blood sugar control. They need to comprehend the risks involved in this diet before deciding whether it's suitable since intermittent fasting may not suit everyone. There is some standard information related to intermittent fasting, followed by meal planning advice, which can aid those starting a regimen involving such practice easily.

Assessing Your Current Health

Before commencing any fasting regimen, diabetic patients must evaluate their current health. Such an evaluation should involve thoroughly assessing the patient's overall physical condition and closely monitoring and comprehending the individual's blood glucose levels. Establishing diabetes management objectives is essential so that satisfactory results can be achieved when intermittent fasting is undertaken; thus, with assistance from a healthcare provider, suitable targets for blood glucose and insulin concentrations can be formulated based on age, sex, activity level, and other relevant factors.

It is of the utmost importance that patients keep a close eye on their physical indicators of overall health, such as weight and heart rate, at every doctor's visit or during periodic checkups with medical professionals. In addition to allowing ample time for restfulness and leisure when initiating intermittent fasting for diabetics, it behooves one to guarantee adequate weekly exercise to stay fit and healthy. Lastly, an honest assessment concerning mental well-being should be performed, too. Mental clarity can surpass physical fitness when trying out intermittent fasting, as partaking in it while overwhelmed or anxious may impede success.

What is the best first meal for intermittent fasting?

Intermittent Fasting has gained fame over the past few years due to its potential to help diabetic patients better regulate their blood sugar levels. Before embarking on this dietary approach, however, proper preparation must take place; this includes making sure you choose the appropriate meal for your first Fast. When utilizing Intermittent Fasting as part of a diet plan, it becomes necessary to consider what type of food is most appropriate when breaking one's fast.

Those engaging in intermittent fasting for diabetes management should consider a light snack high in protein and low in carbohydrates as their ideal first meal. Protein can help suppress hunger and mitigate sudden increases in blood sugar levels. Consuming some healthy fats can also be beneficial because they slow digestion, which keeps you sated over extended periods. Delicious snacks for this approach include:

- Hard-boiled eggs.
- Plain Greek yogurt.

- Cheese sticks.

- Nut-based options such as almonds or cashews.

It is essential not to exceed standard serving sizes when selecting your initial snack while practicing intermittent fasting to manage diabetes; huge servings could make it difficult for one to remain fast until their next mealtime. To ensure food does not impede progress towards reaching target goals concerning insulin levels due to added sugars or artificial sweeteners, opt for only natural ingredients without these components included.

How long can diabetic patients be fasting?

Fasting for a sustained period can be intimidating to diabetic patients, yet it is achievable with the guidance of an experienced medical professional. Awareness of what might transpire and how your body will respond may help make this process more comfortable. The duration one should fast depends on individual metabolic reactions; nonetheless, in general terms, short-term fasting (up to 24 hours) is thought to be secure for most diabetes sufferers. Several research studies have revealed that more extended periods, up to 36 hours, could also improve glucose control and weight management. Consulting with their doctor would likely benefit those considering intermittent fasting or extended-lasting fasts since they are better positioned than others to give personalized advice about appropriate durations based on individual health history and existing diabetes treatment program models. Moreover, through such close contact, regular updates regarding progress during the exercise could be made available, thus allowing any necessary adjustments related to medication dosage to be provided when needed, too.

Medication Review

Medication review is an integral element of the preparation for intermittent fasting among diabetic patients. It is necessary to involve healthcare professionals in this planning process to adjust medications correctly and avoid potential adverse drug effects or interactions. Healthcare providers should monitor glucose levels while assessing how fasting could impact other health conditions, then adjust medications accordingly based on the patient's requirements. Furthermore, individuals must familiarise themselves with any possible interactions between their current drugs and the foods they intend to consume during their fasts. Additionally, patients should ensure they comprehend when to take any crucial medicines while fasting, as these elements might considerably affect blood sugar levels. Besides this, sufferers need to make sure that they communicate openly with healthcare professionals about whatever supplements are taken throughout a fast since some might interact detrimentally with certain medication types. A detailed examination into medicinal use before starting intermittent fasting has scope for setting up patients towards success by eliminating probable dangers that could arise during periods.

Recognizing your type

People with diabetes must be aware of the kind of intermittent fasting that would prove most advantageous to them before embarking on such a plan. By recognizing and distinguishing between various types, individuals can personalize their process for optimal effectiveness according to their needs and tastes. To further facilitate this activity, it is beneficial to take sufficient time to understand diverse types of intermittent fasting and how each type may potentially impact diabetes management. For example, alternating-day fasting (ADF) necessitates eating every other day, while conversely, time-restricted feasting (TRF) demands consumption within predetermined intervals during any given day. Interestingly enough, both methods have been observed to display positive results albeit with discrepancies concerning duration or intensity; thus, it becomes essential that persons enduring diabetes recognize which approach functions best for them so they are able to infer maximum health advantages connected with undertaking sporadic abstinence from food intake.

Health History

It is imperative for those considering the intermittent fasting lifestyle to take their health history into account. It's valid for diabetic patients, who are more susceptible to certain medical complications when undertaking a fast than general populations. Before starting any fasting protocol, it is essential that one consults with a doctor and devises an appropriate plan that considers this individual's particular health profile. It would be prudent in such cases to provide an exhaustive record report, including recent laboratory findings; these should also be updated while engaging in intermittent fasting. Moreover, other pertinent factors like Body Mass Index (BMI), age, symptoms or prior diagnoses related specifically to diabetes, nutrition patterns, etc., must all be considered and taken into account before beginning on your journey towards implementing an intermittent fasting regime. Thus, acquiring all required information beforehand will enable physicians to furnish sound counsel and devise viable treatment strategies if necessary."

Baseline Measurements

Baseline Measurements are of paramount importance for individuals with diabetes who intend to commence intermittent fasting, as they will enable them to monitor their development and make appropriate alterations if necessary. It is recommended that patients evaluate their bodies in three fundamental areas before beginning: glucose levels, body weight, and meal sizes. Glucose levels furnish a baseline signifying how well the person's diabetes is regulated. Body weight measurements provide an indication of pre-fasting energy balance. Meal portion measurements offer information regarding food intake and dietary habits. In addition, Diabetic Patients need to confer with their healthcare provider ensuring that intermittent fasting can be done without any risks given their state and current medications taken. After baseline measurements have been noted down precisely, a plan may be formed that specifies the types of foods that ought to occur during meals before or after the Fast, along with other nutritional regulations or concerns that must be considered accordingly. With these initial observations on hand, Diabetic Patients can begin organizing for intermittent fasting while being certain knowing they possess an outline providing vital clues concerning progress throughout this process.

Setting Realistic Goals

It is essential for diabetic patients starting their intermittent fasting journey to set realistic goals to succeed. Trying to achieve lofty ambitions that are difficult, if not impossible, may cause more harm than good as the individual will likely feel demoralized and disheartened at being unable to reach these objectives. Therefore, they must create achievable targets considering their unique situation and start with baby steps before steadily increasing the level of difficulty involved.

It is essential for those with diabetes who are interested in commencing intermittent fasting to consult a physician before making any dietary changes. It is because blood sugar levels can be subject to drastic shifts when transitioning from one pattern of eating habits into another and, therefore, getting a doctor's advice should guarantee safety and mitigate potential hazards related to nutritional alterations. Moreover, it may also benefit them if they set achievable objectives that allow room for progress over time while still providing a sense of success; this could involve establishing ambitions pertaining to periods without nourishment or consumption, such as endeavoring an objective of abstaining from food intake over 12 hours four days per week or keeping minimal non-carbohydrate snacks between meals. A medical professional might offer helpful guidance about how interim fasting could be tailored based on existing health issues and nutrient requirements.

Consultation with a Healthcare Professional

Diabetic patients must consult with a healthcare professional before initiating intermittent fasting. This consultation can enable them to discuss their medical history and the effects of multiple treatment options on an individual basis, customizing recommendations based on their personal needs, objectives, and lifestyle. Additionally, this dialogue may provide insight into any potential problems that could arise from pursuing intermittent fasting, thereby preventing possible medical risks or complications arising from it. The healthcare provider can help ascertain which type of fasting plan better suits the patient's requirements; they may also supply information regarding likely side-effects associated with it as well as answer any questions posed by the said patient before beginning. Ultimately, such conversations allow individuals greater understanding when attempting healthier habits in accordance with set health goals through intermittent fasting.

General Precautions

Intermittent Fasting, a dietary practice where an individual restricts calorie intake on certain days or for predetermined periods of time, has gained prominence as a way to manage body weight and improve health. Nevertheless, individuals with diabetes should evaluate some crucial aspects before initiating an intermittent fasting diet. They must understand the mechanism behind intermittent fasting and pay attention to which food groups will help them get maximum benefits from it. Moreover, consulting medical professionals such as doctors and nutritionists before beginning a routine of periodic abstention from eating might be prudent advice.

One of the main anxieties for diabetic patients contemplating intermittent fasting is regulating blood sugar levels since they are particularly susceptible to variances in glucose concentrations over 24 hours. It can be resolved by utilizing medication treatments or altering meal timing and ingredients depending on each individual's exclusive requirements. For example, suppose someone inclines hypoglycemia during a fasted state. In that case, it might be advantageous for them to ingest larger meals before beginning the refrained duration to preserve proper blood sugar amounts throughout their day.

It is essential for individuals with diabetes participating in intermittent fasting regimens to select foods that will support optimal glycemic control and guarantee sufficient usage of some micronutrients such as vitamin D, calcium, magnesium, and zinc. Moreover, including fibrous carbohydrates within each meal helps slow digestion while assisting in better glucose regulation. Subsequently, when engaging in an intermittent fasting routine, one must frequently monitor their blood sugar levels so any potential obstacles can be swiftly attended to before they become more serious. Furthermore, gaps between meals should preferably remain within four hours without extended periods of not eating lasting beyond twenty-four hours except under medical supervision, along with advice from a healthcare provider adept at nutrition therapy appropriate for persons with diabetes.

Conclusion

Intermittent fasting can be an excellent tool for those with diabetes to gain better control over their blood sugar levels. It necessitates meticulous meal planning and monitoring, but with the appropriate guidance and knowledge, it can make up a practical element of any program to manage diabetes. With the proper preparation and support system, intermittent fasting may be an uncomplicated yet highly effective way for diabetic patients to work their health properly.

Chapter 6:

Popular Intermittent Fasting Protocols

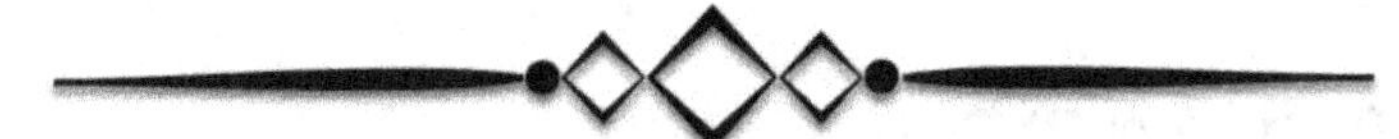

People with diabetes are encouraged to regulate their diets and weight to observe the fluctuations in blood sugar levels. Intermittent fasting protocols have come into prevalence among those with diabetes as a means for facilitating metabolic health and controlling glucose levels. Various forms of intermittent fasting, ranging from time-restricted eating through alternate-day fasting up to Eat-Stop-Eat, can be productive for people with diabetes when adhered to properly. Through an exploration of the diverse types of intermittent fastings available, along with outlining the advantages each method has for diabetic individuals who pursue control over their weight and sugars while still being able to enjoy succulent foods.

The 16/8 Method:

The 16/8 Method, often called the Leangains protocol, has become a popular intermittent fasting plan that many individuals with diabetes have found successful in controlling their condition. This approach involves abstaining from food for sixteen hours continuously each day and consuming all one's meals within eight hours. Rather than demanding drastic calorie limitation, this meal strategy emphasizes selecting times at which snacks and meals are taken to achieve ideal regulation of blood sugar.

A study published in 2018 revealed that when compared to Continuous Energy Restriction (CER) dieting, participants following the 16/8 method encountered significantly more significant decreases in weight, waist circumference, body fat percentage, and triglyceride levels.

Furthermore, this approach has also been demonstrated to help control blood sugar levels. During fasting periods, insulin sensitivity increases due to the release of stored glucose, which gives energy; thus, it can benefit people with diabetes since they do not need medication or injections so often. The 8-hour eating window also allows people with diabetes to have regular meals without overindulging or causing an abrupt spike in their glucose through sugary snacks between these meals. Finally, evidence shows that providing at least 14 hours of fasting daily may reduce inflammation and oxidative stress caused by prolonged elevated blood sugar linked with diabetes.

The 5:2 method:

Intermittent fasting's 5:2 method is becoming popular among individuals who have diabetes. This dietary approach involves consuming drastically reduced calories on two non-consecutive days per week, while average caloric consumption is allowed for the other five days. The advantages of utilizing this program consist of weight loss, increased sensitivity to insulin, and better glycemic control in general. Furthermore, it may also decrease risk factors associated with cardiovascular disease, such as lowering harmful cholesterol levels and augmenting good cholesterol levels.

For those with diabetes, it is essential to consult their healthcare provider before utilizing the 5:2 fasting approach, as an abrupt transition towards a low-calorie diet could cause severe changes in blood glucose levels. Moreover, any alterations of medications must only be undertaken upon the advice of one's physician. Furthermore, consuming adequate nutrient-dense foods during the five "normal" eating days is required for people with diabetes to employ this technique. Intermit fasting may not always suit all individuals due to certain medical conditions or potential medication interactions; thus, it should only be implemented following consultation with a doctor or registered nutritionist while exercising caution and care. Finally, pregnant women and children are advised against such practices since they might more easily suffer from malnutrition than adults when crucial nutrients are absent on reduced-calorie days.

Alternate-Day Fasting

Alternate-day fasting is a favored intermittent fast protocol for people with diabetes. It necessitates that individuals engage in abstaining from food or consuming just insignificant calories on their alternate days. In contrast, they consume between one-fourth to one-third of their everyday caloric needs on non-fasting days. This practice gives rise to periods when insulin concentrations remain low, thus contributing to better glucose regulation among people with diabetes. Research has confirmed the beneficial effects associated with alternate-day fasting, such as reduced blood sugar levels, improved HbA1c, and body weight parameters related to diabetes management.

While this method may be unfitting for specific individuals, those who can conform appropriately could reap its benefits as an approach involving restricted calorie intake. Before initiating any form of fasting, interested parties should receive guidance from health specialists to guarantee safety standards and appropriate nutrition status are maintained throughout the process.

Time-Restricted Eating

Time-restricted eating is becoming an increasingly popular intermittent fasting protocol among individuals with diabetes. The primary principle of this technique consists of consuming one's daily calories within a set timeframe, commonly 8 or 10 hours. Doing so permits 16 or 14-hour periods for fasting between meals and snacks. When conducted properly, time-restricted eating can improve blood sugar levels and decrease insulin sensitivity by allowing the body to rest amid meals rather than being overwhelmed with continual food intake.

Furthermore, one study suggests that fasting on alternate days, including varying amounts of time-restricted eating, could benefit both type 1 and people with type 2 diabetes when practiced under physician supervision. It is essential to consider whether the potential modifications fit into an individual's lifestyle and are safe before beginning any diet changes. It may be prudent to start with shorter fasts (6–8 hours) and gradually increase as needed, paying attention to how the body reacts. Additionally, people who have diabetes should aim at dispersing their daily calorie intake throughout the day rather than partaking in a single large meal. As a rule of thumb, this strategy should be employed multiple times per week but only on non-consecutive days.

Combining Intermittent Fasting Protocols

Intermittent Fasting is a prevalent way to manage blood sugar and insulin levels for persons with diabetes. It involves sustained periods without eating, followed by food consumption within designated temporal spaces. By restricting one's intake to certain hours, regulating glucose concentrations within the body can be possible. Moreover, when combining intermittent fasting protocols alongside dietary adjustments, further health benefits may become accessible in people with diabetes; these might include avoiding processed foods wholly or partially reducing added sugars and simple carbohydrates while increasing their daily intake of whole items such as fruits, vegetables, and lean protein sources. As a result of this conjunctional regimen concerning nutrition management among diabetic individuals, they potentially could gain better control over their insulin concentrations while experiencing higher degrees of welfare overall.

Scientific Perspective

From a scientific standpoint, intermittent fasting has been proven to be an efficient means of diabetes management. Several studies have examined its effects on health outcomes in those with type 1 and 2 diabetes. One study found that individuals who have Type 1 Diabetes saw improvements in their glycemic control after merely two weeks of intermittent fasting.

Additionally, a systematic review involving multiple studies determined that all forms of time-restricted eating can help lower one's fasting glucose levels and strengthen overall glycemic regulation for people affected by Type 2 Diabetes. Moreover, another study suggested that intermittent abstinence may abate inflammation amongst patients who have Type 2 Diabetes -- which is quite often seen as a side effect related to this condition -- while also causing positive alterations in one's body weight. Owing to these findings, it has now become acknowledged as a practical dietary approach towards managing each respective type of diabetes successfully, thereby opening up possibilities regarding further research into its efficacy when employed over more extended periods within lifestyle interventions.

Safety and Considerations

When considering intermittent fasting protocols for diabetics, safety and apposite considerations are of the utmost importance. Individuals with diabetes who participate in physical activity may benefit from some form of intermittent fasting; however, they should be conscious of the potential risks accompanying any specified fast. One such risk is hypoglycemia or low blood sugar levels, as individuals with diabetes have a predisposition to experiencing rapid declines in their glucose levels, which necessitates close monitoring while partaking in intermittent fasting.

Individuals with diabetes who intend to follow a fasting protocol must consult their healthcare provider before starting intermittent fasting. Moreover, they should discuss any modifications in the meal plan or insulin regimen with them. Furthermore, for those already possessing a medical condition or taking medications, it is especially significant to obtain educational advice from an expert healthcare professional before embarking on any new dietary regime that involves extended periods without consuming food.

Due to personal health conditions and diets varying wildly amongst different people, what may be beneficial for one person might not be successful for another. As such, numerous approaches can be taken when seeking out the best intermittent fasting protocol suitable for someone living with diabetes; these will incorporate differing lengths of time between meals and fasts together with distinguishing types of foods eaten during every phase - as such, getting acquainted closely with all available options beforehand proves essential while deciding upon an appropriate program tailored towards individual needs.

Conclusion

Intermittent fasting has become increasingly common among those with diabetes as it can assist in managing blood sugar levels and decrease the potential for long-term complications. There are four distinct fasting protocols: time-restricted eating, alternate-day fasting, eat-stop-eat, and the five two diets. While further research is needed to determine which type of intermittent fasting regimen provides the optimal benefit for diabetics, many individuals have reported positive consequences from engaging in some form of prearranged abstinence from food intake regularly. Before initiating any interval fast plan, one should consult a physician regarding all relevant questions they may have concerning this practice.

Chapter 7:

Healthy Meals for Intermittent Fasting

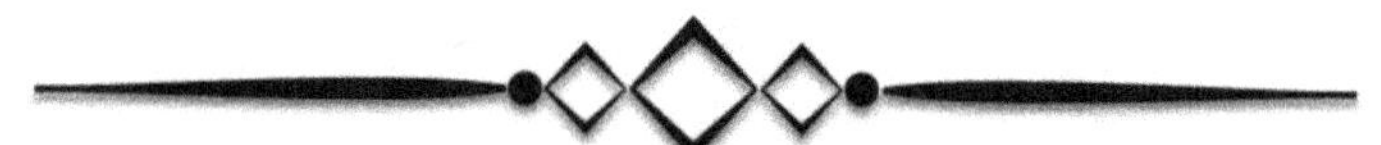

Integrating intermittent fasting into your lifestyle to achieve better health and physical condition is the ideal spot for you. Here, we discuss Healthy Meals about Intermittent Fasting and a selection of recipes and meal plans designed to familiarize individuals with healthy nutrition. From snacks before fasting periods down to meals post-fasting times, our cooking ideas guarantee satisfaction. Furthermore, advice regarding creating meal plans relevant to one's habits and objectives can also be found here.

Importance of Balanced Meals during IF

It is essential to consume balanced meals during Intermittent Fasting (IF) for the body to receive the nutrients that promote proper functioning and support energy levels. Eating an assortment of nutrient-rich food, such as fruits, vegetables, lean meats and seafood, nuts and seeds, whole grains, legumes, and healthy blubbers like avocados or olive oil should be included when fasting. Consuming well-balanced meals guarantees your body adequate vitamins, minerals, and compounds known as antioxidants, which can help protect against diseases.

Eating balanced meals is also essential for promoting healthy digestion; prioritizing consuming fiber-rich foods can help ensure regularity throughout an individual's journey with intermittent fasting. Further, having a diet comprised of balanced meals while using Intermittent Fasting may result in better regulation of blood sugar levels than those consisting primarily of processed carbohydrates and refined sugars. Moreover, it is critical to include adequate amounts of protein into one's eating regimen when intermittently fasting so that muscle mass can be retained; however, care must also be taken not to consume proteins during this time lest weight gain occurs excessively. Every person is unique; thus, the best approach will vary depending on personal preference before starting with Intermittent Fasting. Consequently, consulting empaneled healthcare professionals beforehand helps guarantee appropriateness for each case situation and provides optimal health benefits by weaving balanced meal choices within such regimens.

Different IF Protocols (e.g., 16/8, 5:2, OMAD)

Intermittent fasting is a dieting method that involves alternating between periods of eating and abstention from food, either within the same day or over an extended duration. During this time frame, people can utilize various IF protocols - including 16/8 protocol, 5:2 protocol, and OMAD (one meal a day). When used wisely, these approaches offer numerous health benefits - such as optimizing body composition to improve insulin sensitivity and hormone balance. Nevertheless, consuming nutritious meals during the fasting period is critical for these advantages to be realized. Consuming too many unhealthy foods while intermittent fasting may increase weight due to a heightened caloric intake.

It is essential to be mindful of the nutritional quality of food ingested during periods when engaging in intermittent fasting. A balanced diet that contains lean proteins, healthy fats, complex carbohydrates, and fiber-rich fare will ensure an adequate energy supply without causing blood sugar levels to surge. Moreover, guaranteeing sufficient hydration by drinking plenty of water daily while complying with an intermittent fasting regimen should benefit cognitive functioning and physical performance over fasted intervals.

How IF Affects Metabolism?

The impacts of intermittent fasting (IF) on metabolism are determined mainly by the macros and calorie consumption rate. For IF to bring about any tangible outcome, it is required for the body to have a caloric deficit, meaning that fewer calories must be consumed as compared with those utilized throughout the day. In this fashion, the body is compelled to enter "starvation mode," whereby stored fat will be burned off for energy rather than relying heavily upon everyday intake of food items. Moreover, most versions of IF necessitate changing when meals are taken and what edibles constitute them. Intermittent fasting has demonstrated itself capable of inducing substantial rises in metabolic rate, which assists one's system in burning more calories even while at restfulness. It becomes particularly efficacious if coupled with physical activity such as weight lifting or running, encouraging muscle growth while enhancing metabolic functionality. Furthermore, lower levels of sugar plus refined carbohydrates included within diets governed by IF often lead individuals to display lessened hunger cravings, thus making it simpler to adhere diligently towards their plan and reducing the general amount consumed through intake daily calorific hierarchy.

Balanced Meal Planning for Intermittent Fasting:

A balanced meal plan for intermittent fasting is essential to sustaining optimal health. Macronutrients are crucial when considering the dietary requirements for intermittent fasting, therefore receiving special attention and consideration. Properly dividing these foundational nutrients - proteins, carbohydrates, and fats - is desirable to achieve an excellent ratio to facilitate better digestion and improve daily energy levels.

Micronutrients such as vitamins and minerals are vital for maintaining health during this type of fasting since they supply the necessary nutrients the body requires to function optimally. Consuming a variety of nutrient-rich whole foods will guarantee that these micronutrients can be easily accessed. It is also crucial to consider the significance of hydration during this form of fasting, considering that sufficient water uptake helps foster numerous metabolic processes within the body. Incorporating several glasses of plain or flavored water at every meal may assist in guaranteeing that one's body is provided with ample fluids regularly.

Low Glycemic Index Foods in IF

Nutritionists are increasingly recommending the utilization of low glycemic index (GI) foods when it comes to adhering to an intermittent fasting diet, as these kinds of food can help quell unhealthy surges in blood sugar levels. Food items with a GI rating of 55 or lower are well-known for being low GI and commonly contain high amounts of dietary fiber and protein. When ingested during periods when one is following an intermittent fasting lifestyle, they assist in reducing hunger pangs and forestalling energy lapses caused by unexpected plunges in blood sugar concentrations. Slow-burning carbohydrates like fruits, vegetables, wholegrain breads, and oats must be consumed regularly. Including beans and lentils alongside other legumes in one's daily nutrition intake serves another beneficial purpose: ensuring that complex carbohydrates form part of the menu while keeping GI values within acceptable boundaries. Low GI edibles supply durable vigor while sustaining satiety longer than high GI sources, e.g., cakes, candy bars, and sugary drinks, comparatively speaking. Furthermore, using fibrous fruits plus veggies similar to apples or broccoli will aid in activating regulating hormones, enabling improved control over eating habits throughout the day.

Meal Examples for Fasting Days

One of the most widely adopted varieties of intermittent fasting is 16:8, in which a person observes periods of abstention from nourishment lasting sixteen hours daily and consumes all their food within eight hours. Those who have chosen this protocol for implementing intermittent fasts must replenish with nutritionally dense meals sufficient to sustain them until their upcoming mealtime. Consequently, what are some excellent examples of such sustenance when beginning one's new regime? Breakfast on a day dedicated to fasting may comprise oatmeal crowned with fresh berries accompanied by almond butter and honey.

Oatmeal is abundant in fiber, which assists with keeping a feeling of fullness for an extended period while offering carbohydrates and protein to be utilized as energy. Berries contain antioxidants that help decrease inflammation and boost one's immune system. Almond butter paired with honey provides healthy fats along with natural sweetness.

Moreover, another nutritious breakfast option can be a smoothie of fresh spinach or kale, banana, almond milk, or coconut milk combined with blended flaxseed or chia seeds. Smoothies are highly nourishing and may be prepared beforehand to save time when the morning starts abruptly. Kale and spinach are highly beneficial sources of vitamins A, C, E, and K, folate, calcium, iron, magnesium, potassium, phosphorus, and zinc. Furthermore, bananas offer a healthy serving of carbohydrates accompanied by the bonus of vitamins B6 & C and fiber, while flaxseeds contribute wholesome omega-3 fatty acids to one's meal. Regarding lunch on a fasting day, it could be suggested that one make a salad topped with grilled chicken breast or tofu.

Salads are an ideal way to incorporate much nutrition into one meal. As for the base, lettuce, such as romaine or baby spinach, is suggested, while tomatoes, onions, and peppers can be used as topping along with other vegetables according to personal preference. It is recommended that dressings like olive oil, lemon juice, tahini, and maple syrup be used instead of traditional options. To further augment its nutritional value, this meal should include concentrated protein sources, such as grilled chicken breast or tofu, to keep hunger at bay between meals. These examples provide only a small sample size from which nutritious dishes may be selected during intermittent fasting; nevertheless, there exists a large variety depending on individual tastes – therefore, an assortment of ingredients ought to be tried until desired results occur.

Meal Examples for Non-Fasting Days

On non-fasting days, individuals need to plan their meals in a manner that allows them to access essential nutrients and ensure a balanced diet. It is beneficial for most people to strive towards having meals comprising at least

25 grams of fiber, 20-30 grams of protein, and an array of colorful fruits and vegetables while being mindful when considering how many calories are consumed. Despite individual goals varying from person to person, this type of meal planning can be used generally by anyone looking to provide enough nutrition and fuel the body correctly.

Examples of healthy meals on non-fasting days may include:

- Breakfast burritos with eggs, black beans, and bell pepper.
- Tuna salads with quinoa, celery, and cucumber.
- Grilled chicken sandwiches paired with mixed greens.
- Black bean burgers topped with guacamole and tomato.

Salads made from fresh vegetables such as spinach, kale, and Brussels sprouts combined well with omelets or frittatas composed of scrambled eggs, or egg whites can offer a nutritious option for lunchtime fare. Additionally, snacks, such as nut butter spread onto whole grain crackers, provide an easy way to stay sated between meals. Ultimately, ensuring adequate nutrition during non-fasting periods helps offset fasting intervals and prevent exhaustion caused by nutrient deficiency over time.

Sample Meal Plans

Intermittent Fasting (IF) is a widely embraced approach to diet and nutrition that can provide multiple health benefits. Meal plans are an essential part of IF, as they aid in keeping track of the amount of food being taken in and guaranteeing the correct types of foods have been consumed. Some examples of meal plans designed specifically for people practicing IF involve a 16/8 Intermittent Fasting Plan, a 5:2 Intermittent Fasting Plan, and an OMAD (One Meal A Day) Intermittent fasting plan. Specifically, the 16/8 intermittent fasting plan requires consumption during eight hours followed by sixteen hours fasted throughout any given day."

During the eating period, individuals can consume three or two larger meals, which have been divided throughout the day depending on personal preference. The plan also recommends consuming nutrient-dense foods such as seedy protein sources such as fish and chicken and healthy fats including olive oil and avocados at every mealtime. Additionally, unprocessed fruits, vegetables, whole grains, and dairy products should be included when following this diet regimen. As for the 5:2 Intermittent Fasting Plan (IF), there are two non-consecutive days where food intake is limited to just 500 calories per day while maintaining the balanced nutrition principles outlined previously.

On days other than those where fasting is followed, individuals should adhere to their favored diet with no restrictions on caloric intake. This approach works best when practiced intermittently instead of consistently throughout the week due to its degree of intensity.

Ultimately, OMAD involves consuming all daily calories within a single-hour window without any limitations regarding the types of food consumed. Foods suggested under this plan are similar to those advised in other IF programs;

nevertheless, care must be taken so that essential nutrients such as proteins, carbohydrates, and healthy fats are ingested during each meal. People who practice this plan may discover that tracking calories or resorting to an online nutritional calculator can be advantageous aids when arranging meals that meet their specific needs while remaining beneath the calorie limit mandated by OMAD standards.

Tips for Success

Knowledge of one's dietary needs and preferences is the initial step in constructing a meal plan for intermittent fasting, which can be fruitful if done correctly. It is important to pick foods right for you and eat them at suitable times. Here are some suggestions on how best to accomplish this:

When selecting meals, one should prioritize nutrient-dense options such as lean proteins, complex carbohydrates, healthy fats, fruits, and vegetables for the body to receive all necessary vitamins, minerals, and other nutrients throughout the day. Furthermore, adequate dietary fiber must be included so satiation is achieved on fewer calories when following intermittent fasting protocols; fiber helps slow digestion, which then maintains blood sugar levels for more balanced energy production. Moreover, drinking plenty of water should be remembered since proper hydration keeps hunger pangs away and ensures maximum absorption from consumed food sources. Additionally, consideration needs to be taken concerning timing when planning these meals during intermittent fasting regimes; this usually requires eating window restrictively within 8-12 hour intervals only each day - thus, most calorically dense foods ought to be consumed early morning hours instead while leaving light snacks late afternoon/evening before bedtime rest becomes due. An organized plan can ultimately guarantee success with any dietary program, including periodic fasts.

Conclusion

Intermittent fasting can be a highly advantageous method to enhance overall health and well-being. By meticulously organizing meals and finding healthy recipes designed for this purpose, it is possible to integrate periodic abstinence from food into one's lifestyle with desirable results. With some research, anyone can identify the correct regimen that best suits their needs. Consequently, if someone wishes to supplement their sporadic fasting program with beneficial nourishment components, now is an opportune moment to search through all available options.

Chapter 8:

The Role of Exercise in Blood Sugar Management

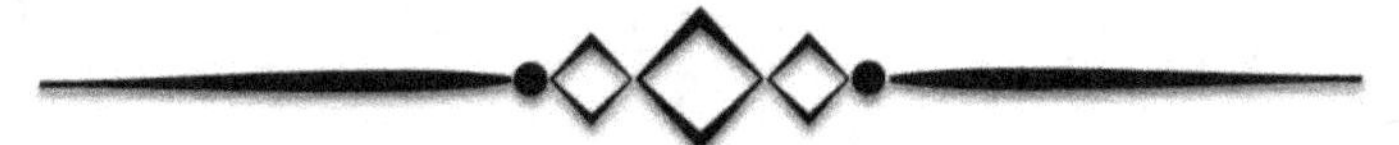

Exercising is integral to managing one's blood sugar levels and preventing diabetes. For diabetics, in addition to being at risk for developing type 2 diabetes, there must be attention paid to their blood sugar levels and the effect on overall health. Exercise plays a significant role in controlling one's blood glucose level and reducing the probability of complications related to diabetes. We will see how exercise can be utilized to help oversee your blood sugar levels while sustaining a sound way of life with this condition and provide some advice about what activities are most beneficial for individuals who have diabetes; additionally, we describe methods that exercising into daily living could be easily incorporated without compromising on controlling one's blood glucose level.

Importance of Blood Sugar Management

Blood sugar management is a significant factor in overall health and well-being. Exercising has the potential to be an essential part of assisting individuals in sustaining healthy blood sugar levels. Regular physical activity can aid in boosting insulin sensitivity, thereby reducing the quantity of insulin required for shifting glucose into cells and decreasing the likelihood of developing type 2 diabetes. Additionally, regular exercise may reduce body fat, which is also associated with blood sugar levels.

Furthermore, when combined with a balanced diet, exercise enables individuals to successfully manage their weight, which has been associated with an improved ability to control blood sugar levels. Moreover, physical activity heightens energy and reduces fatigue, which tends to be connected with abnormally low or elevated glucose in the bloodstream. For those who already have diabetes, regular exercise is essential for maintaining healthy blood glucose concentrations. When done consistently, it can help reduce A1C - a measure used for evaluating average glycemia over a two-to-three-month period -which provides people with diabetes with information on how effectively they are dealing with their illness. Nevertheless, even considering all of these advantages, it is still essential for people controlling blood sugar through changes in dietary habits and exercising regimens to speak first about this matter with their medical advisor before initiating any alterations concerning wellness perceptions or lifestyle preferences.

Benefits of Regular Exercise for Blood Sugar Management

Exercise is a significant factor in controlling blood sugar levels and promoting better general well-being. It can lower the likelihood of developing diabetes or other ailments and decrease the necessity for treatment in those already diagnosed with diabetes or any condition requiring glucose regulation. Regular exercise confers numerous advantages to individuals in adjusting their blood sugar levels.

To begin with, engaging in physical activity can augment insulin sensitivity, allowing cells greater capacity to use insulin proficiently so that they may move glucose from one's bloodstream into individual cells."

Additionally, exercising invokes the breakdown of glycogen stores into glucose, which delivers a source of energy for cells without necessitating further input from the body's existing insulin reserve. Furthermore, exercise can also result in higher production of antioxidants; these chemicals mitigate cell damage caused by chronic inflammation associated with high blood sugar levels and thereby improve cardiovascular health through lessening plaque accumulation in arteries and an overall decrease in inflammation across organs within the body. It may also reduce the possibility of cognitive deterioration due to long-term elevated atherogenic LDL cholesterol concentrations. Finally, regular physical activity application renders psychological advantages such as declined stress levels and improved sleep habits - essential factors when managing consistent glucose levels for an extended duration. Exercise can bring about heightened self-belief and better control over dietary selections that sustain healthy glycaemic homeostasis.

Types of Exercises for Diabetes

Regular exercise has been demonstrated to provide a beneficial effect for those with diabetes, appearing to be able to improve blood sugar control. The selection of practices can also be essential in maintaining healthy glucose levels. Aerobic activities are recommended for people suffering from this condition since they contribute effectively towards burning carbohydrates and increasing the body's sensitivity to insulin. Additionally, strength training is advantageous because it can help build muscle, which works as energy storage. Flexibility and balance exercises may help diabetes patients enhance their mobility along with reducing the risk of accidents or injuries occurring during physical activity sessions; moreover, High-Intensity Interval Training (HIIT) also provides many benefits specifically tailored toward individuals living with diabetes, such as fat reduction and increased metabolic rate efficiency. Considering all types of exercise available that enable physiological and psychological well-being among those affected by the disorder - it is noteworthy that these should form part of any comprehensive treatment approach suggested for diabetic patients.

Creating an Exercise Routine for Blood Sugar Management

Constructing an exercise regimen to oversee blood sugar is vital for anybody with diabetes or pre-diabetes. It has been established that physical movement can diminish glucose levels in the body and enhance insulin affectability. Customary physical action can likewise help a person shed pounds, which is critical for individuals who are large or hefty and experience difficulty overseeing their blood sugar degrees. A custom-fitted activity routine can be altered to suit an individual's necessities by considering age, well-being condition, way of life, and some other applicable elements.

The advantages of exerting oneself for someone with diabetes or pre-diabetes can be manifold, including improved insulin sensitivity, augmented energy expenditure, and better blood glucose control in general. Furthermore, it has the potential to decrease cholesterol levels while diminishing the possibility of developing cardiovascular disease. Moderate-intensity aerobic activities such as walking, jogging, swimming, cycling, dancing, and tennis are all shrewd decisions for individuals with either diabetes or pre-diabetes. Strength training exercises may also be beneficial as they build muscle mass, positively impacting insulin sensitivity.

You must consult a healthcare professional first to create an exercise drill tailored to your needs. It will enable them to assess your health condition and suggest the most appropriate type of physical activity. After identifying what fitness regimen is suitable, it becomes essential to set attainable goals that can serve as encouragement in maintaining your regular workouts over time.

Establishing objectives that one can reasonably accomplish, such as attending three classes per week at the gym or going on a daily walk, may assist in making one's routine more agreeable and maintainable over the long haul. It is likewise fundamental that before participating in any physical activity, you properly warm up so as not to overexert muscles or hurt oneself further; this could be done by stretching before starting any exercise regimen. Moreover, it is suggested that short breaks should be taken during physical activity sessions if required; this aids with avoiding weariness while still keeping up ideal execution during the workout session itself. Lastly, always drink plenty of water during physical activities beforehand, amidst, and after exercises since lack of hydration can prompt tiredness, which meddles with security and performance amid workout sessions.

Overcoming Challenges and Staying Motivated

Exercising can be highly beneficial for those regulating their blood glucose levels. Being active assists in keeping stable and healthy glycemic numbers, yet staying persistent is only sometimes uncomplicated. Achieving success in this undertaking necessitates the identification of any difficulties that may impede the establishment or maintenance of an exercise regimen; these could diverge person by person and might include physical impediments engendered by medical conditions, deplorably limited time allotment, as well as just plain lack of interest or prompting.

It can be challenging for distinct individuals to discover an exercise program that they appreciate and can proceed with over time. One potential solution is to attempt various activities until a positive association emerges between the individual and the action itself. Even basic physical exercises such as walking, swimming, or cycling have been documented as advantageous in supporting long-term blood sugar regulation, provided it is done chronically. Determining which of these applies to an individual will assist them in making their upcoming steps more achievable.

A further hindrance that people frequently encounter is the need for additional motivation beyond simply controlling their health condition. Establishing reasonable objectives and remunerating oneself when they are accomplished can aid in building positive reinforcement that encourages further involvement. It is also vital to recall that not every workout needs extensive duration; even modest physical activities performed steadily suffice for most individuals and conveniently fit into occupied timetables without interference. Though these impediments might appear daunting initially, taking the needed time and effort shall yield rewards in improved glucose control over an extended period. With regular exercise comes success--and assurance knowing one is doing all possible for overall well-being!

Safety Considerations

Exercise has been long-acknowledged as an efficacious means of regulating blood sugar levels. However, other significant elements must be considered when exercising for this purpose. Safety must always come first and foremost in any situation. Those with diabetes must evaluate their fitness level before commencing a new exercise program, as intense activity could evoke either too low or too high glucose levels from the diabetic individual. Furthermore, it is essential that upon exercising, one monitors their blood sugar regularly.

Taking the necessary precautions to avoid injury and maintain proper hydration while engaging in physical activity is prudent. Conversation with a doctor about an appropriate level of intensity should be sought by individuals wishing to exercise safely, as excessive exertion can put persons at risk for hypoglycaemic episodes or other health complications. In addition, any sudden changes in blood sugar levels must immediately be brought before a medical expert for appraisal and further counsel on how best to cautiously adjust the frequency and strength of exercise.

Hydration and Nutrition

Hydration and nutrition are both indispensable components in controlling blood sugar. In any exercise program, it is imperative to remain sufficiently hydrated during workouts and over the day so that fatigue and dehydration, which may result in low blood sugar levels, can be prevented. Additionally, it is critical to supply the body with its required nutrients before, while undertaking, and post-workout. Eating a bite-sized snack before exercising helps guarantee that energy levels are upheld while providing supplemental fuel for an effective workout. During physical activity, replenishing fluids and electrolytes dissipated because of perspiration aids in preventing dehydration. After exercise, consuming healthy carbohydrates assists in reviving muscle glycogen levels, concurrently helping govern blood sugars that this exertion could have influenced.

The Future of Diabetes Management with Exercise

Exercise has been revealed to possess various advantages in managing diabetes. By selecting an appropriate form of exercise, someone with diabetes may enhance overall wellness while controlling their blood glucose levels. Evidence suggests that exercising boosts insulin sensitivity, which aids in monitoring sugar concentration and prevents conditions such as neuropathy and kidney harm. Furthermore, engaging regularly in physical activity can help those who have diabetes reduce their dosages of medication – mainly if a nutritious diet plan accompanies it. It should also be noted that routine exertion might lower one's chance of developing type 2 Diabetes for individuals who are genetically inclined or overweight, respectively.

When constructing an exercise program for a person with diabetes, certain factors should be considered:

1. All activities undertaken are recommended to have a moderate intensity level to ensure no health risks are posed by over-exertion.

2. Adequate hydration and regular monitoring of blood glucose levels before starting physical activity and during and after its conclusion should also be observed.

3. Having something sugary on hand at all times would help significantly if one's blood sugar suddenly decreases, either while exercising or shortly afterward.

The future looks promising for those managing their diabetes due to recent technological developments and healthcare treatments intended for this purpose. Exercise remains highly beneficial when included within any regimen designed specifically for individuals living with diabetes; improving overall well-being while reducing potential complications associated with uncontrolled changes in blood sugar values achieved through consistent efforts within such practice regimes could very likely result from such actionable measures indeed revolutionizing how we presently view long-term efficacy vis-à-vis lifestyle modifications enacted today, without doubt, carries excellent promise down the road.

Conclusion

Exercise is an essential element in managing blood glucose for those with diabetes. Regular physical activity assists in controlling sugar levels even when insulin and diet are insufficient. A mixture of aerobic exercise, strength training, and stretching can help foster healthy sugars and decrease the chances of long-term problems associated with diabetes. With a balanced eating regimen and regular workout program, individuals diagnosed with this condition may be better equipped to handle it and live healthier lifestyles.

Chapter 9:

Combining Intermittent Fasting with Exercise

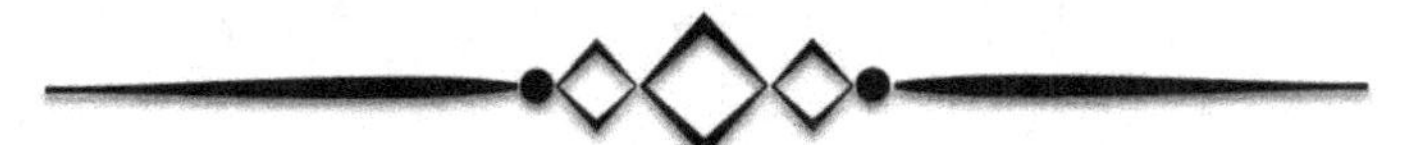

Intermittent fasting combined with exercise could be the solution for you! Recent years have seen intermittent fasting grow in popularity as an efficient weight-loss method, but it also presents plenty of benefits for people with diabetes. With regular exercise taken into account, too, intermittent fasting can assist in controlling one's blood sugar levels and promote healthier living standards. Combining these practical strategies can help those suffering from diabetes to keep their health intact while managing their glucose levels successfully. Can such methods make life less complicated? How beneficial are they? We will discuss all these factors.

Intermittent Fasting Basics

Fasting is a fashionable diet regimen that involves switching between eating and not consuming. It's generally done by stuffing yourself for a precise amount of time, usually 8 hours per day, then fasting the rest of the day. Alternatively, folk can go without food for 2-3 days before resuming regular diets the subsequent week. The inference behind intermittent fasting is that it may be helpful when trying to shed weight and provide potential health advantages such as improved blood sugar control and lessened inflammation – but does this work?

For lots of people with diabetes, combining exercise with intermittent fasting could be a helpful way to take care of their condition. It's no surprise that diabetes is increasingly common nowadays - which means people are searching for new ways to monitor their glucose levels, like dieting. Joining fasting with working out takes away any uncertainty regarding controlling carbohydrate intake - something different folks affected by diabetes have difficulty doing every day and wondering if this approach might work well enough for you. Why not ask your doctor about it? In addition, cycling between eating and fasting periods can help reduce insulin resistance - commonly found in those with diabetes – leading to improved glucose metabolism over time. Exercise also plays a vital role in helping one regulate blood glucose levels as it helps the body use insulin more effectively and increases sensitivity. To make full use of intermittent fasting and exercise for better management of diabetes, people with diabetes could create a program alternating short bursts of intense physical activity with longer breaks where they would do rest or low-intensity activities such as walking or light jogging. In this way, these two elements combined may help improve control over their condition long-term.

Timing Meals Around Workouts

When it comes to people with diabetes, they need to pay extra attention when looking after their blood sugar levels. Mixing intermittent fasting and exercise is vital to guarantee that these remain in the healthy range. Planning snack or meal times around physical activity can be a great way of keeping your glucose under control. So this should be something for people with diabetes think about doing beforehand.

They need to create an overall plan that includes both workout sessions and eating patterns; by following what you have planned out carefully, you will get all the benefits from fasting fitfully and regular exercising together.

It's crucial for those with diabetes to time their meals according to when they're going to exercise. Eating a snack or meal before getting physical will help level out blood sugar and give them energy during the workout. Once it's over, having something again helps fill up the body's fuel stores as well as helping muscles recover from exertion better through nutrients. Skipping meals before or after working out can be damaging due to its effect of altering glucose levels - plus, there isn't enough sustenance either while doing exercises or afterward during the recovery period.

When planning your food schedule around exercising times, considering serving size and carbohydrate type ahead is paramount; likewise, you need snacks containing proteins and complex carbs like fruits & whole grain bread post-workout. Hydration is another essential point — dehydration leads not only to lower glucose counts but subsequent exhaustion, insufficient concentration & raised chances of hypoglycemic episodes, too. What is the way around this? It's best practice to drink plenty of water daily whether you plan on training or otherwise.

Pre-Workout Nutrition

Regarding pre-workout nourishment for diabetics, the amount and timing of food consumed before exercising can significantly affect your performance and general well-being. Intermittent fasting is sometimes prescribed to control blood sugar levels in those with diabetes, but combining this with exercise may be tricky. It's worth emphasizing that everyone has individual reactions to different foods and metabolic rates – so you should speak to an authorized nutritionist or medical professional before making any significant changes - after all, we want our fitness journey to be safe!

Considering pre-workout nutrition is essential if you're an intermittent faster or a diabetic, here are some general tips for most people. For physical activities lasting longer than 30 minutes, your body needs carbohydrates to work at its best - and this means eating around

30 to 60g of carbs two hours before any exercise. The right choice would be choosing food sources such as whole grains, fruit, and starchy vegetables – all good options!

Alternatively, you might have a small snack (such as a banana) 15 minutes before exercising; this could be particularly helpful if you've only got limited time or need an extra boost during the session. It's essential to ensure you're adequately hydrated with water depending on several factors, such as how warm it is outside and your energy levels - but don't forget to keep topped up not just before working out but also while exercising and afterward for ideal fluid balance. For protein intake, aim for 20-30g of each meal beforehand; this can help power muscle development by supplying our body with the necessary amino acids. Good options include lean meats like chicken & turkey breast, fish including salmon or tuna, and plant sources of proteins like beans or lentils. Lastly, although fats may seem contradictory when trying to reach weight loss objectives, they are essential for hormone creation; incorporate healthy alternatives such as nuts & seeds in moderation within an hour before starting your workout routine.

During-Workout Strategies

Exercising is essential for those with diabetes to get glucose into the cells and use it as energy. It can be hard to balance exercise and food when managing your blood sugar levels; however, combining intermittent fasting with workouts makes this easier. Strategies surrounding exercising are essential for people with diabetes because their blood glucose can change at an accelerated speed due to physical activity. People should also remember that intense or long-term exercises may cause tiredness, appetite cravings, and thirst, which must be managed carefully during these times.

It can lead to quite a drop in blood sugar levels, which might cause hypoglycemia (low blood sugar). If this is not dealt with satisfactorily, it could result in dizziness, confusion, and even passing out or coma based on how severe the low blood sugar situation is. Knowing when and what you should eat before an activity, as well as during it, is very significant for anyone managing diabetes who works out regularly. How do I ensure optimum energy while exercising? Can my body handle long periods without any food intake before exercise? These questions should be considered if one wants their workout session to go smoothly.

A great way to pair intermittent fasting with exercise is having a light snack before your workout session if you haven't eaten for over eight hours; this should ensure your energy stays at the right level by giving some extra glucose. A small helping of protein foods like a hard-boiled egg or yogurt combined with complex carbohydrates such as whole grain breads or fruits can provide enough energy without overly affecting your insulin levels. How awesome would it be to gain all these advantages while still sticking to our diet plan?

Research also suggests that having low glycemic index (GI) foods 45 minutes before doing exercise may prevent potential falls in blood sugar during activities - examples include oatmeal, peas, and lentils; these have less of an impact on your insulin levels when compared with other higher GI food such as white bread and sweet treats. Also essential is drinking fluids containing electrolytes throughout the workout session plus regular glucose testing; this gives you greater control over any changes taking place so that immediate action can be taken if required.

All in all, combining intermittent fasting and exercising can benefit people with diabetes. Still, it's paramount to get the right strategies into practice at suitable times: eating smaller meals full of complex carbohydrates before working out and keeping tabs regularly. At the same time, training should help avoid sudden drops in blood sugars occurring while exercising, which could lead to different health issues if left unchecked.

Post-Workout Nutrition

If you're after combining intermittent fasting with exercise, post-workout nutrition is as essential for people with diabetes as it is for everyone else. Eating foods loaded with protein and carbohydrates immediately following a workout can help protect against muscle tissue harm and refuel the body's energy stores before your fast commences. Protein helps to mend cells while boosting metabolism; carbs replenish glycogen levels. For those of us living with diabetes, opting for low glycemic index food options whenever practical aids in keeping healthy glucose levels - have you found what works best?

After you've got your sweat on, fueling up is essential. A small bowl of oatmeal or granola with fruit is a great post-workout snack, as is yogurt with fresh berries and nuts or even a hard-boiled egg with some whole-grain toast. Macronutrients are essential here - aim for around 20g of protein and 30-50g of complex carbs. Balance this out nicely without overloading the portion size too much. Your body will feel depleted after all that exercise, so whatever you eat should get absorbed quickly into the bloodstream, leading to raised blood glucose levels if not careful - yikes. Remember hydration, too; replenishing those fluids lost during physical activity is essential, so get rid of guzzling down plenty of water afterward.

Special Considerations

Regarding intermittent fasting for diabetics, some matters warrant particular attention. Above all else, you should chat with your doctor or dietician before adjusting your diet. It is essential if the change involves not eating anything for long spells; someone with diabetes must understand how their body will react when taking such an extreme dietary route, as this could cause fluctuations in blood sugar levels. Before beginning any kind of fast, you must adequately research what type of approach you're about to follow - after all, knowing what it entails can make a huge difference!

No two people with diabetes are the same, so any protocol must be tailored accordingly. Depending on how severe one's diagnosis is, specific protocols may not even be safe for those who suffer from pre-existing conditions or take particular medications - expert advice is essential here. When it comes to exercise while intermittently fasting, again, you must get a doctor or a certified trainer before embarking on anything new; exercise has been shown to help handle blood sugar levels and improve insulin sensitivity, but too much can cause them to crash quickly! Some individuals prefer more frequent meals as fuel leading up to their workouts, while others could benefit from having food immediately after training sessions to stop further drops later. There isn't a 'one size fits all' for diabetics (or anyone!) trying out intermittent fasting alongside exercising: understanding your body's unique response beforehand will save possible trouble ahead — wise words indeed!

Practical Tips and Guidelines

When managing diabetes, exercise and intermittent fasting can be a potent combination. People with diabetes must understand how to create an enjoyable yet safe routine that incorporates both practices. To ensure your safety while doing this, you should always talk with your physician or healthcare provider before planning any exercises. Here are some practical tips and guidelines that could help when combining intermittent fasting with training for people living with the condition:

To begin, one of the most critical things is checking your blood sugar levels before getting physical activity started and after - making sure everything has settled back down again afterward; something essential if you want all efforts not to go in vain.

You must ensure your body is fueled with enough glucose before physical activity - this could mean having a snack first or taking medication. Additionally, please keep track of how long it has been since you last ate and adjust insulin levels accordingly. When scheduling exercise around fasting – if the day requires abstaining from food, more strenuous activities are best done in the morning when blood sugar is still somewhat elevated. For lower intensity things such as walking, we recommend completing these near breaking your fast point for the day.

Whenever you're doing any form of physical activity, it's always wise to have something with natural sugar, like juice or snacks, in your pocket just in case you feel dizzy or drained during exercise. Diabetic people need to fast and

exercise simultaneously intermittently –
dehydration could result in serious health issues
such as a greater risk of heart attack or stroke.

Therefore, those engaging in this lifestyle must
ensure they drink plenty throughout the day
(especially while working out). It should help
maintain their glucose levels steady and prevent
unexpected drops due to hypoglycemia caused
by dehydration. People with diabetes must
monitor their electrolyte balance during long-
term periods without food, which can lead to
further dehydration risks if not monitored
enough.

Conclusion

People with diabetes can benefit from
combining intermittent fasting and exercise to
regulate their blood sugar levels. A balanced
diet and regular physical activity can help

increase insulin sensitivity and improve glycemic control, essential steps toward better diabetes management. What's more, if you time your meals right and pair them with the correct type of exercise, this could have an even more significant impact on glucose metabolism, thus resulting in improved health outcomes overall! So why not give it a go? You've got nothing to lose but plenty to gain.

Chapter 10:

Troubleshooting Challenges

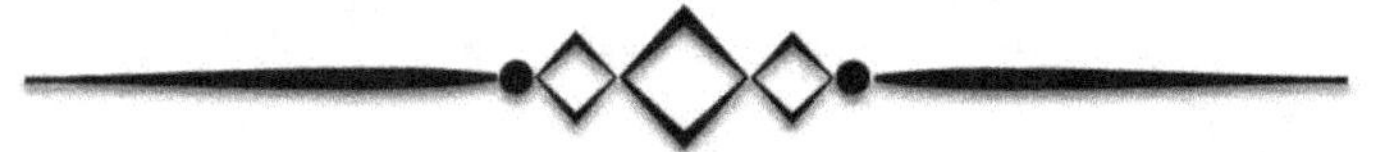

s it hard for you to properly care for your health due to the condition? If so, know that there are others in similar situations. Taking charge of Diabetes can be difficult, and if steps aren't taken to maintain appropriate blood glucose levels, this could result in serious medical issues. Fortunately, several tips and strategies might help those living with Diabetes conquer their troubleshooting challenges. We will explore different aspects associated with managing Diabetes, such as diet control and exercise guidance, among other topics related to the subject matter. Additionally, advice on staying healthy while tackling any troubleshooting obstacles shall be provided herein.

Importance of managing hunger, cravings, and plateaus

Maintaining a beneficial blood sugar level is one of the primary references for individuals with Diabetes. It requires managing hunger, cravings, and plateaus effectively. Hunger in diabetics can be handled by multiple techniques, including preventing it through eating smaller meals or snacks more frequently throughout the day to reduce any discomfort, carefully monitoring carbohydrate intake, keeping hydrated with water, low-calorie beverages, or herbal tea, and increasing consumption of lean proteins such as eggs and fish. Meanwhile, cravings may be managed by finding healthier options instead of sugary items that still offer stimulating flavors while providing satisfaction at the same time. Plateaus are often addressed using exercise, which burns calories but does not cause an increase in glucose levels or adjusting dosages on insulin shots or oral medications taken regularly. Additionally, taking probiotics every day has beneficial effects when looking to maintain balanced levels of blood sugars comparatively, too. All these measures should be used together if people living with diabetes wish their respective glucose readings to remain within acceptable parameters consistently.

Understanding Hunger Pangs

People with diabetes often experience difficulty with hunger pangs, especially those who have type-1 Diabetes. The pancreas cannot generate insulin, which is essential for correctly processing carbohydrates. Without adequate amounts of insulin, carbohydrates cannot be metabolized effectively; therefore, they cannot provide energy to one's body. Consequently, individuals with Diabetes may feel intense hunger pangs even after consuming food. To ward off this discomfort, people with diabetes must understand what triggers these feelings so that correct steps can be taken to treat them. The most prevalent cause behind diabetics' feeling excessively hungry lies within their blood sugar levels dropping too low."

Blood sugar levels that are too low can result in a situation referred to as hypoglycemia, which causes intense feelings of hunger even when the person has recently ingested food. It is paramount for individuals suffering from such an issue to be able to recognize its symptoms and quickly eat something to avoid severe medical problems. Other possible reasons why someone might feel hungry include dehydration or not eating enough due to guilt or dread of gaining weight; both issues should be addressed through lifestyle changes like drinking adequate amounts of water and consuming meals without restrictions or remorse.

It is essential for Diabetics to precisely monitor fluctuations in their blood sugar levels over a day if they are to manage any hunger pangs successfully. Blood sugar meters, uncomplicated gadgets that enable individuals to quickly ascertain their levels to spot developed issues before they become grave hypoglycemia or hyperglycemia, can help them accomplish this task. Furthermore, tracking dietary intake and physical activity may also prove helpful when detecting any patterns or catalysts connected with changes in both blood sugar levels and hunger pangs. With these instruments available, people affected by Diabetes can assume control over creating and following through on an action plan concerning how best to regulate their appetite while averting potential long-term health risks related to uncontrolled Diabetes.

Coping with Hunger Pangs

Individuals living with Diabetes must contend with the persistent challenge of controlling their hunger sensations daily. Proper blood glucose levels can be preserved only when people who suffer from this condition regularly consume meals and snacks between sunrise and sunset. Regrettably, such individuals may often discover that they become hungry at intervals that stand separate from routine meal times; this abrupt hunger could cause steady sugar concentrations to rise too high or drop too low, ultimately causing symptoms like nausea, exhaustion, and other unease.

To combat this issue of staying satiated between meals and snacks without raising blood sugar levels, nutritionists advise several strategies people with diabetes can implement. Ingesting slow-digesting foodstuffs such as beans, nuts, fruits, and vegetables may assist in keeping one feeling full for longer. Additionally, incorporating proteins into each meal or snack helps reduce the rate at which any carbohydrates consumed are digested. Furthermore, regularly drinking copious amounts of water keeps the stomach saturated and staves off cravings for unhealthy or sugary treats.

The most crucial step regarding managing Diabetes is speaking with one's doctor about their dietary requirements based on their situation and lifestyle. They will be able to put together an eating plan that guarantees adequate nourishment while maintaining even blood sugar levels regardless of hunger pangs experienced between mealtimes; understanding how best to control appetite and create nutritionally balanced dishes shall be essential when it comes to assisting people with diabetes to live fulfilling lives despite all difficulties associated with having this illness condition.

Dealing with Cravings

For those battling with Diabetes, cravings may seem like an impossible challenge. It is effortless to succumb to the temptation of irresistible indulgences; however, people with diabetes must take control of their cravings as, without sufficient management, they can have grave implications on blood glucose levels. Therefore, constructing a plan that will help individuals tackle these desires in a secure and balanced manner is essential. Recognizing triggers ought to be the initial step in dealing with yearnings.

Certain types of food may stimulate cravings for some individuals, while intense emotions or social settings come into play for others. Awareness of these triggers can assist people in anticipating prospective problems and making more sensible nutritional selections when faced with attractive snacks.

Discovering alternate methods of coping with stress, such as yoga or exercise, can be particularly advantageous since they provide people with diabetes with healthier avenues to express their feelings and decrease the hazard of succumbing to unhealthy solutions. In addition, maintaining healthy nibbles helps prevent them from grasping sweetened versions when hunger sets in; some decent alternatives include fruits, low-fat yogurt, nuts, and whole grains.

Finally, if desires become too challenging to overlook, people with diabetes must indulge responsibly and guarantee that the portion size remains within recommended instructions; this will avert sudden increases in blood sugar levels without completely relinquishing the pleasure derived from savoring a preferred snack. Ultimately, finding strategies for dealing with difficult situations and incorporating more healthful choices into diet regimes can empower diabetic persons to manage their dietary needs while fulfilling random longings sufficiently.

Strategies for Overcoming Plateaus

People with diabetes often experience Plateaus, during which the condition appears to have stagnated, and treatment is no longer effective. It can be incredibly distressing, particularly when even lifestyle modifications fail to make desired changes. Nevertheless, some tactics may help in overcoming plateaus concerning diabetes management. While some medications have demonstrated efficacy in surpassing a table and should be discussed with a doctor for an individualized strategy, it is also essential to remember that various environmental factors, such as illnesses or stressors, must sometimes be considered. Eating nutritious meals combined with regular physical activity has been known to enhance blood sugar levels potentially, thus enabling advancement past any given plateau state. Finally, yet importantly, consulting healthcare providers before making decisions related to diabetic plateaus would always remain prudent since they will offer invaluable knowledge on how best to tackle these issues while developing plans tailored according to your respective medical history and personal needs.

Conclusion

The management of Diabetes can be a complex process that requires active effort and dedication. To meaningfully address this condition, individuals living with Diabetes must watch their blood glucose levels regularly, carefully manage their diet, and exercise routinely. It is also recommended for those facing challenges related to diabetic complications to seek professional help when necessary. Crafting an action plan consisting of targeted steps may prove beneficial in helping curb potential issues associated with having Diabetes.

Chapter 11:

Monitoring and Tracking

Progress

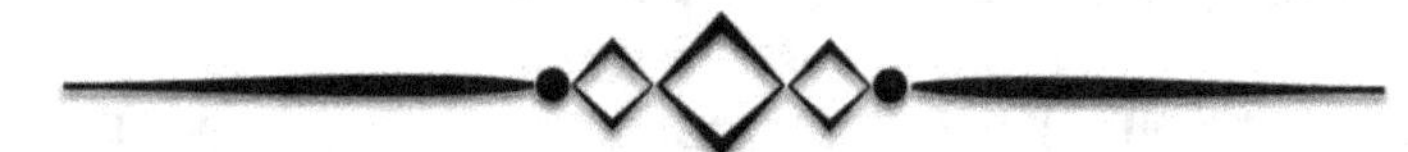

As a person with diabetes, there is an emphasis on managing one's blood sugar levels and overall metabolic health that cannot be understated. Intermittent Fasting has been established as a viable option for such management due to its efficacy being proven in numerous studies; however, the effects of intermittent Fasting, specifically for people with diabetes, remain somewhat unknown. To gain more insight into this subject matter, we will examine the different ways that can assist with tracking progress when using intermittent Fasting as part of diabetes management. We shall consider why it is so vital to monitor and track progress while utilizing intermittent Fasting for diabetes care, along with how best you may go about doing just that.

Tracking Blood Sugar Levels

It is necessary to monitor and track the progress in intermittent Fasting for individuals with diabetes to manage their condition effectively. Amongst all metrics, one that must be vigilantly monitored is blood sugar levels. It will ensure that glucose concentration does not become too high or low, which can cause many major health problems. Tracking the blood sugar level during intermittent Fasting would need to occur before intakes of meals/snacks are made to ensure it does not plummet suddenly or start trending downwards unacceptably low.

It is imperative to pay attention to the amount of insulin taken when measuring blood sugar, as it is frequently administered while fasting so that glucose levels do not exceed normal ranges during periods without food. Keeping tabs on diabetes and adhering to intermittent Fasting can be incredibly helpful in understanding how your body responds and whether any necessary modifications should be made about nutrition or medication use. Monitoring blood glucose is essential for people with diabetes who are following an intermittent fast regime, as this data guides what food items may be consumed and at which intervals these meals should occur.

Keeping a Food Diary

Maintaining a food diary is indispensable in managing diabetes and executing intermittent Fasting. It allows people to trace their dietary consumption. It changes their blood sugar levels throughout the day and assesses behavior patterns in what they eat that could result in elevations or dips in their diabetic symptoms. Keeping a record of meals eaten can also assist individuals with diabetes in staying faithful to eating each day, thus helping them reach objectives for losing weight or restraining glucose amounts. Besides this, it may give an understanding of how particular foods interact with the body's functions and which edibles should be taken more often or less frequently. By engaging oneself into dutifully inputting suppers and snacks into a food journal, people with diabetes can enhance overall healthiness plus monitor any alterations happening within glucose concentrations so one can surmount controlling their ailment over time."

Setting Milestones

Establishing milestones is critical to any intermittent fasting regime for those with diabetes. Setting goals enables an individual to assess their development more precisely and hold themselves responsible for the accomplishment or failure of the diet. Before beginning, it is essential to have realistic, practical milestone expectations that will inspire when achieved. At least weekly weigh-ins should be performed to monitor any weight changes over time, and adjustments may be made accordingly. In addition, blood glucose measurements should also be taken and documented regularly during fasting to guarantee levels stay within conventional limits. Even though reaching each milestone might take longer than anticipated, having these standards present serves as a reminder of why one has adopted this lifestyle change initially. It additionally acts as an affirmation they are being proactive about their health by assuming control of their diabetes through intermittent Fasting.

Combining Blood Sugar Monitoring, Food Diary, and Milestones

For individuals with diabetes, intermittent Fasting can be beneficial in managing blood glucose levels and enhancing general well-being. Nevertheless, monitoring and tracking progress while following an intermittent fasting lifestyle can be challenging. Establishing suitable criteria of achievement by combining the measures of keeping food diary entries together with regularly checking blood sugar levels before meals, after meals, and before going to bed will offer one efficient means for measuring success and ensuring efficacy.

Blood sugar monitors are relatively inexpensive and easily accessible, making it possible for people with diabetes to monitor their levels, if necessary, continuously. The best approach to ensuring that fluctuations in one's blood glucose level due to intermittent Fasting do not occur is by maintaining a food diary; recording all the items consumed will enable one to recognize patterns of what works better than others.

The more information included in the journal - including portion sizes and when food is consumed each day - the more valuable it can be for recognizing any problematic foods or habits that require change. Formulating objectives throughout one's journey to managing diabetes with an intermittent fasting lifestyle can be a source of encouragement and keep track of progress made over time. Goals such as decreasing A1C levels within a certain amount of months or ceasing snacking at night are achievable targets that concentrate effort on specific goals while using intermittent Fasting as part of diabetes management.

Overcoming Challenges and Seeking Professional Guidance

Undertaking intermittent Fasting as a person with diabetes can be an arduous challenge, and one of the primary elements in controlling diabetes is to ensure progress is assessed and measured against objectives. Achieving success concerning Fasting necessitates a multifaceted method encompassing nutrition, exercising, recognizing potential risks, and consulting medical specialists. While dietitians may furnish valuable insight concerning sustenance requirements, consultation with doctors regarding the appropriate type of dietary plan is essential. In addition to supplying beneficial advice on what kind of fasting regimen would work best for their diabetic patients, physicians are also equipped to help with any difficulties that might arise from such activity as hypoglycemia or ketoacidosis. Furthermore, they have access to extensive healthcare records, which could give vital data relating to previous treatment plans that inform someone's journey toward successful abstention from food intake. Knowing professional health personnel has taken time to appraise someone's lifestyle enables them greater contentment when it comes to making decisions about individual well-being.

Celebrating achievements

It is essential for any individual seeking to fulfill their goals that they celebrate accomplishments. This sentiment also applies to intermittent Fasting for people with diabetes; acknowledgment of milestones is a great way to encourage and concentrate on one's objectives. Celebrating minor successes, such as cutting back daily calorie consumption, shedding several pounds, or accomplishing habitual fasting times, can make intermittent Fasting enjoyable and provide the stimulation required for staying unwavering and self-controlled.

Additionally, celebrating these accomplishments can help reframe our attitudes toward the practice, shifting from an arduous task we dread to one that helps us appreciate our progress. It also serves as a powerful reminder of how far we have progressed and further motivates us to remain devoted to our objectives. We sustain our enthusiasm through meaningful rewards such as taking some time for ourselves or indulging in something enjoyable like going out for dinner or watching a movie. We are also better prepared to tackle future goals without feeling overwhelmed.

Conclusion

It is necessary to closely monitor and track progress to manage diabetes through intermittent Fasting effectively. By checking blood sugar levels and other biomarkers of metabolic health, any alterations or changes within the body can be identified before they become hazardous. In this way, people with diabetes can remain secure while engaging with an intermittent fasting plan yet still receive desired outcomes.

Chapter 12:

Intermittent Fasting and Medications

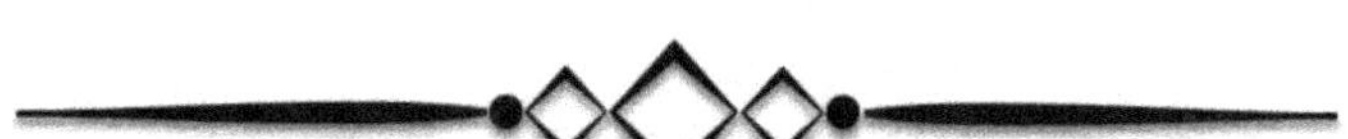

Intermittent fasting has become an increasingly prevalent method of sustaining a healthy lifestyle. Recent studies have evidenced that it is equally capable of effectively controlling diabetes and regulating blood sugar levels. This text shall address the potential advantages of intermittent fasting that those suffering from diabetes may experience, survey various types of drugs at one's disposal, and recommend approaches for combining such treatments alongside medication to achieve ideal diabetic control. We are determined to supply readers with reliable details derived from empirical evidence demonstrating how intermittent fasting can be advantageous when striving towards successful maintenance concerning diabetes management.

Intermittent Fasting and Diabetes

It has been observed that Intermittent Fasting is gaining prominence as a dietary regimen and lifestyle choice throughout the world, with many individuals reporting positive impacts on their health. Recent scientific studies have indicated potential advantages of intermittent fasting for those managing diabetes type 1 or 2. It should be taken into consideration that overall calorie reduction can also lead to improvements in blood sugar levels over time; nevertheless, research indicates there may be beneficial effects connected with insulin sensitivity and glycemic control resulting from intermittent fasting specifically.

Studies have revealed that individuals with Type 1 diabetes who fasted two days per week had lower middle blood sugar levels than those who did not. Moreover, people with Type 2 diabetes experienced an enhancement in insulin sensitivity when they adopted a modified 16:8 approach where their eating window was limited to eight hours, and they abstained from food for the remaining sixteen hours of the day. Researchers are still exploring how intermittent fasting may impact persons with pre-diabetes or metabolic syndrome. It is essential to consult your physician before embarking on any novel dietary program or modifying your current medication regimen while engaging in intermittent fasting.

Adjusting Medication Schedules

The complexity of adjusting medication schedules for intermittent fasting when dealing with diabetes is apparent. Medications may be essential for assisting in controlling glucose levels. Insulin and sulfonylureas are two types of diabetic medicines that can impact the body's natural capacity for regulating blood sugar amounts. Consequently, people with diabetes who practice intermittent fasting must comprehend how their medication affects their system and how they ought to modify their dosage suitably.

Suppose a patient is taking oral medications such as insulin or sulfonylureas. In that case, they may consider reducing their dosage before commencing intermittent fasting because blood sugar levels tend to decrease during this period. A physician can recommend an appropriate dose according to each individual's needs. People with type 1 diabetes may require more guidance; if insufficient insulin doses have been taken before starting the fasts, hypoglycemia or difficulties in controlling blood sugar might result. Conversely, people with type 2 diabetes could choose not to accept specific dosages if their blood sugar remains low during periods of fasting. As no long-term effects are known from making drastic alterations in medication amounts, it is recommended for individuals with diabetes engaging in intermittent fasting to seek advice from medical experts before altering anything.

Types of diabetes medications

Intermittent fasting has garnered increased attraction amongst those searching for ways to better their wellness and accomplish long-term weight diminishment. However, individuals with diabetes must be aware of specific considerations before including intermittent fasting in their lifestyle choices. Principally, the consequences that abstaining from food may have on using medicines for treating diabetes require deliberation. Explicitly speaking, two distinct varieties of medications utilized in diabetic treatment - insulin injections and oral drugs such as metformin and sulfonylureas - should be managed dissimilarly depending upon when an individual initiates a fast.

Typically, insulin is taken in response to or anticipating ingesting food. Individuals with continuous insulin regimens must carefully monitor their blood sugar levels while fasting so they don't experience hypoglycemia due to having low insulin levels combined with the lack of carbohydrates entering their bodies. Moreover, if blood glucose drops too low during a fast for those with Type 1 Diabetes, it becomes necessary to break the fast to prevent possible complications. It thus may not be able to achieve an entire period without eating.

For individuals living with Type 2 Diabetes who are taking insulin, it may be necessary to modify their dosing schedule to prevent the occurrence of hypoglycemia when they engage in fasting. On the other hand, those who take oral medications such as metformin and sulfonylureas as part of their treatment should ensure these drugs are taken right before or during meals for optimal absorption by the body. It is a challenge for those administering intermittent fasts seeking control over diabetes since oral medication must only be consumed following eating activities; thus, persons wishing to pursue this type of fasting ought to speak with a healthcare professional about altering their pharmaceutical regimen before engaging in any prolonged abstinence from food or drastic changes concerning customary feeding habits.

Understanding medication timing and dosages

It is indispensable to understand how insulin functions in modulating blood sugar levels. Insulin reacts to changing glucose concentrations within the bloodstream by triggering cells to take additional glucose out of circulation. By administering a distinct dosage of suitable drugs at an appropriate time, those with diabetes can sustain healthy blood sugar readings.

Interval fasting has become a popular way for people with diabetes to further their health objectives and promote weight loss management; however, one must bear in mind that chronic doses or medications used for treating diabetes may necessitate alteration depending on when somebody decides not to eat food (fast). Persons afflicted with this condition should speak up about intermittent fasting being safe, given any accompanying ailments they have, before modifying to manage their diabetic state.

Factors affecting medication adjustment during intermittent fasting

It is particularly challenging to adjust medications for individuals with diabetes who have chosen to follow intermittent fasting protocols. When determining the best approach, various factors must be considered, including alterations in blood glucose levels, the response of one's body when it comes to food or fasting, and potential side effects due to certain drugs. People taking medication for controlling their diabetes need to closely monitor their symptoms while regularly adjusting medicines to ensure an effective yet safe intermittent fasting regime. An essential factor that has implications for adjusting medications during intermittent fasting is changes in blood glucose levels. When an individual is without sustenance for a prolonged period, their body does not obtain energy from dietary sources. Instead, it relies upon stored energy resources such as fat or glycogen stores. It can result in reduced insulin sensitivity and elevated glucose levels in the bloodstream. Therefore, medications must be adjusted to lower blood glucose while avoiding hypoglycemia or other complications.

The physiological response to the processes associated with intermittent fasting is also relevant regarding adjusting medications during such dietary regimes. For instance, hormones like glucagon-like peptide-1 (GLP-1) are released due to calorie restriction; this hormone assists in regulating glucose levels by conveying information from the pancreas regarding when insulin should be circulated into the bloodstream. Thus, if GLP-1 levels are elevated due to intermittent fasting habits, it may be necessary for individuals on diabetic medicine to have larger doses than usual so that their blood sugar remains within safe parameters.

Moreover, particular types of drugs used for diabetes treatment can produce adverse side effects while intermittently abstaining from eating, given alterations in absorption rates or dosages required throughout lengthy fasts. Consequently, those taking medication prescribed for diabetes ought to consult with their healthcare professional about modifying dosage before commencing any form of intermittent fasting protocol.

Communicating with Your Healthcare Provider

Engaging in an open dialogue with one's healthcare provider is essential if they are pondering utilizing intermittent fasting to manage diabetes. Although many physicians may need to be aware of the concept and scientific basis behind intermittent fasting, those considering this option must come prepared with pertinent information backing their decision-making process. It should also be noted that any medications taken for diabetic purposes must be discussed to discern how such changes in meal times associated with the aforementioned dietary practice will interact in addition to that; furthermore, due to lessened food intake resulting from intermittent fasting, reductions or alterations in medication might become necessary. Therefore, consulting said health care provider ought to provide the most appropriate advice concerning managing prescribed medicines during such period when practiced intermittently. Moreover, periodic checkups by doctors while engaging in interim fasts are paramount for keeping track of blood sugar levels coupled alongside applications specific to it over time; these assessments further enable monitoring progress made therein and deducing whether extra amendments need implementation towards the accomplishment of the desired outcome.

Safety Precautions

The complexity associated with taking medications for diabetes can be extensive. Regarding intermittent fasting and the subsequent administration of drugs, caution is necessary; this has been further complicated by the need to carefully consider timing when determining both efficacy and safety outcomes. Thus, to effectively manage diabetes through intermittent fasting interventions, practitioners must have a comprehensive understanding of different classes of diabetic drugs and an insight into their intricacies.

Individuals with diabetes should always exercise caution when considering intermittent fasting. Insulin dosage must be adjusted according to changes in glucose levels and monitored regularly. Furthermore, those taking oral medication must either consume the dose alongside food or forgo it on days when no meal is finished so as not to increase their risk of hypoglycemia. Those doing an extended fast lasting more than twenty-four hours may require additional medical supervision due to fluctuations during that period.

People with diabetes must understand what healthcare providers recommend regarding medications taken while engaging in intermittent fasting and consult a certified Diabetes Educator (CDE) who can give tailored advice, thus ensuring personal needs are met while remaining safe throughout such activities. Despite potential risks associated with the consumption of certain medicines under these conditions, they can generally be managed if guidelines suggested by healthcare professionals are followed conscientiously.

Hypoglycemia prevention and management

It has been proposed that intermittent fasting may help with diabetes, and preventing and managing hypoglycemia is significant. Hypoglycemia can be brought about by numerous factors, including medications prescribed for diabetes, if not regulated carefully. Eating multiple meals throughout the day is an efficient approach to keeping stable glucose concentrations to lower the risk of hypoglycemia. Intermittent fasting also assists in preserving consistent glucose readings since it involves periods when you consume food, as well as times when there are no intakes (known as fasts). During these intervals, your body will utilize its stored energy sources instead of depending on dietary intake to uphold regular glucose amounts. In addition, it is necessary to monitor your blood sugar when taking any medication for people with diabetes before changing what you eat or medicine dosages; thus, ensuring safe and effective management against hypoglycemia must always be consulted with health providers first."

Emergency protocols

People with diabetes should take their medication precisely as prescribed and with the utmost vigilance, particularly when combined with intermittent fasting. For those suffering from diabetes, it is essential to have emergency protocols in place to guarantee they receive the requisite medical assistance if glucose levels become low or high during fasting. Emergency protocol standards exist for both hypoglycemia and hyperglycemia. Hypoglycemic states are constituted by blood sugar below 70 milligrams per deciliter (mg/dl), while a level of 180 mg/dl comprises hyperglycemia.

It is of the utmost importance for people with diabetes to adhere strictly to their doctor's directions and become well-versed in suggested procedures in an emergency. Concerning hypoglycemia, it is paramount that immediate action be taken so as not to allow serious health consequences to occur. An individual displaying signs of hypoglycemia should ingest 15-20 grams of rapid-acting carbohydrates such as juice or candy to back up their blood sugar levels into an acceptable measure. If, after fifteen minutes, indications are still prevalent, then more portions of carbohydrate must be ingested until manifestations dissipate entirely.

It is recommended that patients carry glucagon kits to self-administer in the event of a severe episode of hypoglycemia requiring help from another person for recovery. In cases of hyperglycemia, it may be necessary to lower insulin dosage or take supplemental oral medications designed to diminish glucose levels in the bloodstream. Depending on the severity, hospitalization could be required if symptoms include confusion or other indications pointing towards ketoacidosis (a state resulting from insufficient insulin that leads to excessive body acidity). If so, intravenous fluids, including electrolytes, can be rehydrated. Patients should consult with their doctor regarding appropriate emergency protocols and how they might adjust medication during intermittent fasting periods when needed.

Conclusion

Intermittent fasting is gaining traction to regulate blood glucose levels and administrating medications for diabetes. Research demonstrates numerous potential advantages to fasting in managing this condition, including augmented insulin sensitivity, enhanced body composition, decreased inflammation, and lower concentrations of hemoglobin A1C. Although further research needs to be conducted on the long-term implications fasting has for controlling diabetes effectively, current evidence suggests it can be an invaluable tool when dealing with diabetic medication administration and stabilizing sugar content within the bloodstream.

Chapter 13:

Long-term Health and Wellness

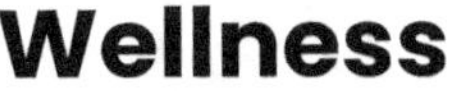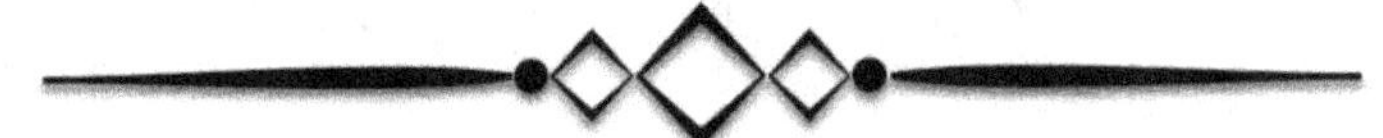

Intermittent fasting might be an answer for unlocking a healthier, sustainable lifestyle. It endeavors to explain the concept of intermittent fasting and how it can offer protection from getting afflicted with diabetes and other health complications. The potential advantages regarding wellness resulting from intermittent fasting will be discussed in this section, along with any conceivable risks attached should one decide to follow such a way of life. Moreover, we shall investigate how incorporating such practice into daily activities may bring benefits.

The importance of long-term health and wellness

The importance of long-term health and wellness cannot be overstated, particularly relevant to conditions such as diabetes. Focusing on comprehensive well-being for the longer term has many advantages, most notably in helping prevent the development of intricacies related to diabetes. It is partially attributable to lifestyle modifications triggered by a sustained commitment toward priority personal health endeavors. Such modifications include:

- Substituting healthier diets.
- Ascending physical activity levels.
- Moderating stress intensity.
- Introducing intermittent fasting into customary habits.

It has been ascertained that intermittent fasting plays a crucial role in assisting those with diabetes to ward off any difficulties linked to this disorder. When allowed into one's regimen accurately, periodic abstaining may lead to positive physiological changes such as increased insulin sensitivity, which can diminish the prospect of disabling conditions like cardiovascular problems and cerebrovascular accidents. Moreover, this type of dieting could be beneficial for regulating glucose metabolism among existing diabetics by providing an additional form of protection against possible complications deriving from their condition. Furthermore, certain studies imply that even other chronic diseases like Alzheimer's are subject to some advantages due to intermittent fasting, given its ability to reduce inflammation within the body systemically.

Then, multiple benefits exist correlated with emphasizing long-term well-being while simultaneously permitting requisite periods of abstinence into one's routine lifestyle habits. For individuals diagnosed with diabetes or vulnerable to developing it, carrying out these strategies might prove particularly advantageous in avoiding potential life-altering repercussions connected with such ailments.

Understanding Diabetes and Its Complications for Wellness

Diabetes is one of the most widely experienced chronic illnesses around the globe. An estimated 25.8 million children and adults in the United States have been diagnosed with this condition, with approximately 1.7 million new cases identified annually. Diabetes arises when a person's cells cannot efficiently employ glucose, thus causing excessive amounts of it in their bloodstream. Generally speaking, there are two primary forms that diabetes can take: type 1 and type 2 diabetes - both having distinct characteristics and related negative ramifications associated with them.

Regarding diabetes-associated difficulties, there is a broad scope of potential issues that can result from long-haul hyperglycemia. These include enhanced vulnerability to cardiovascular illness, stroke, renal disappointment, visual impairment, neuropathy (nerve harm), inadequate injury recuperating, and foot ulcers because of nerve harm or fringe conduit sickness (PAD). Intermittent fasting has become progressively well-known for improving insulin affectability and lessening aggravation markers related to ceaseless conditions like diabetes. It includes taking sporadic breaks from eating – such as for 16 hours per day – while concentrating on supplement-thick dinners during admission periods. Exploration has proposed that occasional fasting may have possible advantages regarding improved hazard factors connected with metabolic issues like diabetes; notwithstanding this, additional research should be done to comprehend its impacts over more drawn-out timeframes completely.

Lifestyle Factors in Diabetes Prevention and Management

Various lifestyle factors may contribute to preventing or managing diabetes, being relevant for those wishing to lead healthier lives. Exercise, diet, and stress management are all essential for long-term health in individuals with the condition now or at risk of having it later. Physical activity regularly helps reduce insulin resistance by reducing body fat levels while also building up tolerance towards glucose.

The American Diabetes Association proposes that those who have type 2 diabetes ought to begin an aerobic exercise program, lasting for at least 150 minutes per week, along with strength training two or more days weekly. Furthermore, dietary modifications can also be effective in managing the symptoms of diabetes and preventing further complications; such changes include limiting the intake of sugar products, abstaining from processed foodstuffs, consuming healthy fats like olive oil, and augmenting the consumption of fiber-dense fruits and vegetables.

Adhering to a balanced diet is critical for overall health, yet intermittent fasting has been studied for its potential advantage in controlling glucose levels among those with type 2 diabetes. By limiting caloric consumption on specific days of the week, people might be better able to regulate their sugar measurements when combined with healthy dietary practices. Moreover, tension management should be considered as it can substantially increase blood sugar concentration if left unchecked. Mindfulness exercises such as yoga and meditation may provide calming effects, potentially upgrading glycemic regulation eventually. Lifestyle elements are fundamental to preventing and coping with diabetic implications; physical activity, nutrition, and strain moderation must all be part of one's everyday regimen to attain optimal well-being.

Intermittent Fasting: An Overview

It is increasingly common for individuals to engage in Intermittent Fasting, a dietary practice that involves alternating between times of consuming food and caloric drinks and abstaining from them. This type of fasting can be implemented through Daily Time-Restricted Eating (TRF), where people eat within 12 - 20 hours every day, or Weeklong Fasts, wherein they have one meal per day or consume meals sporadically throughout the week. Compared to more conventional practices such as Calorie Restriction or Macronutrient Manipulation, intermittent fasting has been proposed as having potential health benefits, which makes it attractive.

It has been suggested that the metabolic flexibility provided by intermittent fasting may assist in preventing Type 2 diabetes and its resulting complications. Moreover, research reveals potential benefits for cardiovascular disease danger factors, including cholesterol levels and blood pressure readings. It is also proposed that intermittent fasting might reduce body fat accumulation; however, limited scientific evidence confirms these claims. Some studies suggest it could enhance specific individuals' cognitive performance and mood stabilization.

Although this information is available, one must be aware of a few risks connected to intermittently fasting before following such an approach diet plan: most notably, those suffering from pre-existing medical conditions ought to take precautions when trying any form of fast as doing so without consulting their physician first can lead further health problems or worsen existing symptoms due to interactions with medications taken simultaneously - plus too frequent changes in energy availability during periods of abstinence have the capacity cause imbalances within hormones leading likely result in excessive stress on bodily systems if done incorrectly.

Intermittent Fasting and Diabetes Management

Intermittent Fasting (IF) has grown in popularity recently due to its various suggested health benefits. It has also become the focus of increased scientific research about potential effects on diabetes management. Diabetes is a severe medical condition capable of resulting in life-threatening consequences, including cardiovascular disease and kidney damage.

Evidence implies that Intermittent Fasting can be a beneficial tool for managing diabetes by helping lower blood sugar levels and augment insulin sensitivity. It has been recommended that incorporating Intermittent Fasting (IF) into lifestyle habits may be beneficial to those already analyzed with pre-diabetes or type 2 diabetes and individuals at greater risk of being afflicted by this disease. While the research on such potential benefits is still in its early stages, some studies have indicated improvements in glucose tolerance and insulin sensitivity if short-term IF interventions are undertaken.

Additionally, people who practice intermittent fasting could potentially enjoy other positive effects, including weight loss, improvement in mood levels, and improved sleep quality; however, anyone considering taking up an intermittent fasting routine should first speak with their healthcare provider - especially if they suffer from any pre-existing medical conditions – since long term health must not rely exclusively on one single factor like periodic fasts. Still, multiple components, including medications and alterations to lifestyle habits, would need to play a role.

Implementing Intermittent Fasting Safely

The popularity of Intermittent Fasting has been increasing steadily, especially its potential for enhancing long-term health and mitigating diabetes-related problems. Nevertheless, it is essential to appreciate that while the practice can be beneficial in numerous ways, caution should still be exercised when adhering to it. Therefore, one should only embark on an intermittent fasting regimen if there is expert guidance from a medical practitioner or certified nutritionist who could verify safety and effectiveness and advise on minimizing any negative repercussions.

Furthermore, individuals ought to guarantee that they are still taking sufficient nutrients to satisfy their dietary necessities and provide the body with the necessary fuel for proper functioning. Those partaking in intermittent fasting should strive to concentrate on consuming nutrient-rich foods high in fiber, vitamins, minerals, and antioxidants. Additionally, it is significant to pay attention to hydration levels by drinking copious quantities of water all through the day and careful attention to signs such as headaches or dizziness, which could indicate dehydration.

Finally, managing stress levels proves essential for successful practice within intermittent fasting since cortisol needs to remain balanced so that the body can sustain homeostasis while taking advantage of intermittent fasting practices.

Long-Term Wellness and Sustainability

Fostering long-term health and wellness to hinder diabetic complications is a significant challenge. Intermittent fasting may lend assistance in achieving this mission. When assessing intermittent fasting for diabetes management, two primary facets need consideration: the short-term benefits, which can aid in controlling current blood sugar levels, and the long-term benefits, indicating sustained overall well-being over time, potentially providing an enduring atmosphere for successful diabetes administration. Regarding protracted well-being, intermittent abstaining has been linked to increased insulin sensitivity alongside advanced glucose tolerance.

It has been established that when more insulin is secreted in response to glucose intake, it is effective for better performance; as a result of this increased effectiveness, those individuals at risk of developing type 2 diabetes may help from reduced chances. Moreover, intermittent fasting has also been linked to further protecting against obesity-related metabolic complications. Its heightened metabolic efficiency offers potential advantages such as improved weight loss outcomes through dieting and exercise regimens, decreased cholesterol levels, and other indicators associated with poor cardiovascular health. In addition to these benefits, research points towards its positive impact on memory formation and cognitive functions provided that it is performed consistently over extended periods. At the same time, additional studies are needed to conclusively verify or deny any statements regarding the consequences of intermittent fasting on long-term health results and overall integrity and health. Early indications indicate that there could be efficacy in implementing this approach for combating problems relating to diabetes prevention effects.

Maintaining motivation and discipline

Sustaining motivation and discipline is fundamental in a lengthy health and wellness regimen. Establishing new habits can be challenging, but it's the only means to ensure lasting accomplishments. One strategy is setting incremental, attainable goals. Think about the final destination, break down the steps to achieve it, and then take each action gradually. In addition, locating activities that render adhering to the program effortless also proves significant.

Motivation and discipline are key components to successfully incorporate a long-term health and wellness routine into one's lifestyle; however, consistency will ultimately lead to positive results. To motivate oneself further, incorporating interval runs into the weekly schedule may prove beneficial if running is particularly interesting. Not only will this provide all the advantages associated with intermittent fasting, but it can also be seen as an exciting aerobic workout that provides something to look forward to. Additionally, having someone with similar objectives in mind would serve well as an accountability partner or support system when willpower starts waning. This person could act as a cheerleader, offering encouragement when needed so progress remains on track toward reaching desired goals.

Case Studies and Success Stories

Case studies and success stories are valuable resources for healthcare professionals, researchers, and people searching for information on sustained health management. Especially helpful in understanding how intermittent fasting could help prevent diabetes-related issues such as kidney damage, erectile dysfunction, and nerve damage is the case study approach. One analysis of 15 individuals with type 2 diabetes discovered that despite being prescribed similar medicines, participants experienced improved blood sugar levels due to intermittent fasting. Moreover, indicators of renal well-being were notably higher in those who had followed a fast regimen than those who hadn't. Other research has similarly pointed toward affirmative results regarding glucose control enhancement and metabolic biomarkers related to unhealthy outcomes, corroborating its value as part of an extended health plan, perhaps reducing risks associated with developing diabetic-linked complications over time through intermittent fasting.

Conclusion

It can be seen that intermittent fasting is a constructive approach to long-term health and well-being concerning diabetes prevention. Not only does this practice provide effective deterrence from the potential complications of diabetes, but it also grants considerable wellness advantages that assist in sustaining general good health. Specifically for those already dealing with diabetes, research has indicated that intermittent fasting may offer benefits such as better control over sugar levels and lessened dependence on insulin medication.